BEST DETOX SMOOTHIE RECIPES

10 Day Green Smoothie Cleanse-Lose Up to 10 Pounds in 10 Days!

ASHLEY David

ABOUT THE BOOK

The numbers on the scale and how we feel inside out while staring on these ever increasing numbers…This is the story of countless women around the world and there seems to be so many solutions but they hardly work. This book is all about a practical approach to tackle your weight loss problem without disturbing your work and routine. This solution simply asks you to add the nutrients and vitamins you lack through green smoothies. Adding smoothies to your diet is a wonderful way of nourishing your body with fiber, vitamins and minerals you might not be getting from your diet.

Sometimes, you are told to go on a calorie restricting diet but it doesn't work for everyone. It makes you more frustrated, hungry and you crave more junk food. Green smoothies, on the other hand, are filling and nourishing. You don't feel hungry all the time and the best part is that they actually help you to lose weight. Being a woman, it feels great when you are energetic, your health improves, you can spend more time with friends and family and you can buy those gorgeous form fitting dresses that you adore!

This book provides you with a plan to lose 10 pounds in 10 days. It sounds impossible but it's not if you believe in what you are doing. The first step is always hard but you can fight your hunger and cravings. Add delicious green smoothies to detox your body from all the toxics that have been piling up in your body for a long time. There are 50 delicious, quick and easy recipes you can follow without any difficulty to lose weight and balance everything in your body.

It's not just word of mouth or mere advice, the benefits of these smoothies are obvious as they are made with natural ingredients. They work better than any expensive supplements you buy and they don't have any side effects. The only thing you need is a blender and you can try all these healthy smoothie recipes! Little changes like getting up early, some exercise and drinking smoothies will go a long way in keeping you fit and elevating your self-confidence. Go ahead and take control of your life. You need to do this for yourself and your loved ones.

Table of Contents

INTRODUCTION

Welcome to this exciting and new journey in which you can cleanse and detox your body from all those harmful things your body doesn't need. Our biggest concern today is that markets are loaded with all the attractive and processed foods that are advertised in such a way that we buy and eat them. The results are obvious: we put on excess weight that we can't seem to put off in any way. It's a frustrating and emotionally draining experience.

Many of us are struggling to get our hands on some sort of magical solution to it. There are loads of diets, exercises, lifestyle changes and techniques but the problem is: you can't try everything. So, which one really works? It all boils down to the fact: how can you manage the new diet and lifestyle in the long run. Is it doing anything? Are you finding it difficult to keep track of what you are doing? If you don't have any positive answers to these questions, then you need a better strategy. What is simpler than drinking a glass of smoothie? You don't need to go into minute details like micro and macronutrients, keeping count of calories, etc.

The 10-day detox will be hard for sure but it will be worth it when you lose 10 pounds in 10 days! Plus, you get to try 50 amazing green smoothie recipes that will not only detox your body and boost your energy but help you to achieve the ultimate goal of losing weight. Be confident and start your journey of *10 Day Green Smoothie Cleanse*. The results might blow you away when you see yourself after this challenging transformation.

Switch from your regular meals to drinking healthy green smoothies for 10 days. Consider it a new start for your overall health and fitness. To keep yourself motivated, think about why you started in the first place. Snack on crunchy vegetables, a handful of nuts, apples and some other snacks mentioned in the book when you are hungry. This will definitely curb your cravings and you will feel full and satisfied throughout the day. No hunger! That's an amazing feeling to have when you are on this cleanse. You might feel bored and angry when you see other people eating proper meals. That's where you need to have self-control and remind yourself that it's only for 10 days. This 10 day Green Smoothie Cleanse will help you lose 10 pounds in 10 days. Don't worry! This book will be your guide through this difficult yet fruitful journey.

To give you a more clear idea about this Green Smoothie Cleanse, you should know why it's important for you. The first step in losing weight is to detox your body from the toxic overload that piles up inside fat cells. That is why it's tricky and hard to lose weight through traditional dieting. An effective weight loss strategy not only focuses on fat loss but also on your overall health and fitness. When you complete this cleanse, your body will restore the much needed balance. The combination of green veggies and fruits will heal and nourish your body, making you more energetic than you ever were. The best result besides weight loss is that you will actually enjoy healthy foods. You will not crave all the junk that you liked before this cleanse.

If you want to be completely sure whether you should sign up for this challenge or not, take this little quiz and decide for yourself:

- Do you crave sugar, sweets and processed carbs often?
- Do you eat a lot of processed and fast food?
- Do you drink coffee and tea more than two times a day?
- Do you drink a lot of sodas?
- Do you drink less than 8 glasses of water every day?
- Are you more prone to different infections and diseases?
- Are you sensitive to environmental toxins?
- Are you stressed out most of the time?
- Do you have trouble getting good sleep?
- Do you frequently experience digestive problems like bloating and indigestion?

If your answer is 'yes' to most of these common questions, you might need to take a break from your usual lifestyle habits. You can significantly benefit from this 10 Day Green Smoothie Cleanse.

This book is about how you can prepare your body for losing more weight if you need to. It doesn't leave you hanging after 10 days. Read on to find out how you can stay fit after completing the 10 day cleanse. It will also guide you about maintaining a healthy lifestyle that is not difficult to manage. You will not only get to try 10 different smoothie recipes for 10 days, this book offers you 50 more delicious smoothie recipes that will help you in the long run. We have such busy lifestyles that we rarely have time to make proper healthy meals for ourselves. Making smoothies using fruits and vegetables is an easier way of getting what you miss in your diet. You don't need to buy supplements or go into the complicated scientific details to stay fit. Make your life simple, happy and healthy!

❖ ❖ ❖

CHAPTER 1

What you need to know about Green Smoothie Cleanse?

Naturally, the first question that comes to mind before committing yourself to anything is: What is it all about? The basics of anything matter the most. 10 Day Green Smoothie Cleanse is a way of detoxing your body by drinking green smoothies for 10 days. You will need to drink healthy and nourishing green smoothies instead of eating your regular meals. The thought of giving up regular meals for green smoothies seems hard but that is how you can kick start your metabolism and flush out the all the toxics from your body.

According to this plan, you need to reboot your system. When you start drinking the nourishing and satisfying smoothies, rich in fiber, iron, minerals and vitamins, you provide your body with everything it needs. These smoothies also keep you hydrated and energetic all day. The most common health benefits you will notice after 10 days are weight loss, increased energy levels, better sleep and better digestion. This detox program works wonders for your digestive system and you feel less bloated.

Basic Guidelines:

- The first thing is quantity. You will need to drink 2 liters which is around 14 glasses of smoothies every day. Make your smoothies for the whole day. Keep them in the fridge. Drink a glass at an interval of 4 hours throughout the day.

- You can have healthy snacks too! Eat cucumbers, celery, carrots and other crunchy vegetables you like. If you miss eating fruits, you can have apples. You can also eat high-protein snacks like a handful of unsalted nuts, plain Greek yoghurt, hard boiled eggs and peanut butter.

- Drinking at least 8 glasses of water is a must. Herbal teas are also good.
- Foods that are NOT ALLOWED include meat, white sugar, all the processed carbs, coffee, alcohol, and sodas.

Why do you NEED the Cleanse?

The essence of this 10 Day Green Smoothie Cleanse is to clean your system from everything you have been putting in it. Some say that you don't need any detox plan because liver and kidneys help in clearing out toxins. Surely they do but sometimes it's difficult for our body to process and clean the overload of toxins we are exposed to every day. That is where you need that system reboot. Drinking green smoothies not only flushes out harmful waste, it also restores balance to your body. You are drawn towards healthy food and you feel that you are in control of your cravings.

After going through this 10 day transformation, you will be in control of your health. You will be able to make better food choices and you will like the taste of healthy food. You don't need any expensive and complicated diet plan. All you need to do is, go through the 10 Day Green Smoothie Cleanse and cut out all the bad foods that have harmed your fitness. Enjoy the natural and healthy foods along with scrumptious smoothies. It is a much more practical and easier lifestyle.

How do you know that your body has excess toxins? This is an important question. The answer lies in these symptoms: bloating, indigestion, fatigue, allergies, chronic pain, and infections. Now, these symptoms on their own are not usually connected to the toxins in our bodies. However, they are caused by many lifestyle and environmental factors. So, excess toxins and these health issues do have some relation with each other. We usually take medicine and hope that it will be okay. It gets better but we never make changes in our diet to combat these health issues. Now, doctors worldwide know that half of our wellbeing depends on our diet and the other half on medication in most health conditions and diseases.

The excess toxins are stored in our fat cells which are difficult to break down. The more toxins build up in our bodies, the heavier we get. So, you need an effective detox strategy to clean your system first and then you can lose weight. Vegetables and fruits have healing properties and a lot of health benefits. On top of that, smoothies keep you hydrated which makes it easier to lose weight without feeling weak.

Reasons behind Using Green Smoothies!

Leafy green vegetables are the most important ingredient in these detox smoothies. Their health benefits are numerous. Looking at only a few of them will give you a clear idea why green smoothies are the best option in this 10 day green smoothie cleanse.

Pack a Punch of Micronutrients

Leafy green vegetables pack a punch of minerals, vitamins and phytonutrients. They are rich in vitamins C and E which are very important in preventing cancer. Vitamin B and folate contribute to heart health and prevent birth defects. Ladies! Note this if you want healthy babies.

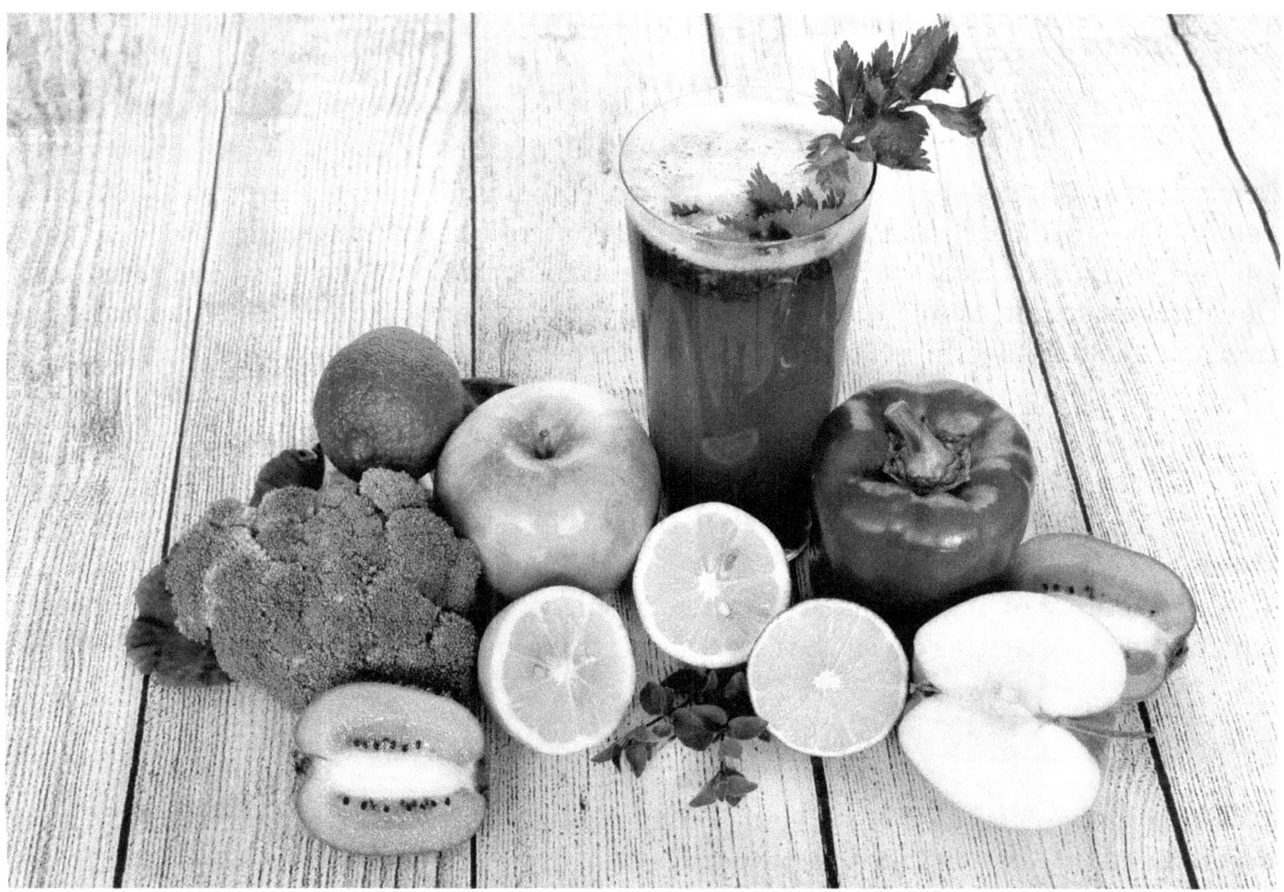

Besides vitamins, leafy greens are rich in minerals like calcium, iron, potassium and magnesium. Without getting into too much detail, all these minerals play an important role in our bodies. Calcium is important for bone health, iron is essential for making hemoglobin and potassium is needed for a healthy heart. Magnesium boosts your immune system and it helps in managing diabetes, pregnancy and menopause.

Fiber:

Leafy greens have loads of insoluble fiber. If you don't know the importance of fiber, let me tell you that it helps in digesting your food and absorbing the nutrients you need. It may sound odd that it's one of those healthy things you can't digest. It helps in improving bowel movement and pushes the waste out of your body. Note that among other things, fiber in your smoothies will help in the detox.

If you are facing problems like constipation, nausea, weight gain and high blood pressure, you seriously need a lot of fiber in your diet. What's better and easier than having a yummy glass of green smoothie! Adding fruits like apples, pears and blackberries along with green veggies like kale or beet leaves will be more beneficial.

Keeps you Hydrated:

Drinking green smoothies will keep you hydrated and fulfill your dietary needs. This will help ease flow of blood in the vessels that will ward off two health issues: high blood pressure and formation of clots in the blood vessels. Green smoothies will also improve your excretion mechanisms, in simple words, you will not face problems like kidney stones, constipation and bladder infections. Staying hydrated is the best way of removing toxics from the body.

Antioxidants

Leafy greens are rich in antioxidants like beta-carotene, vitamins C and E, and minerals. The high content of plant pigments like zeaxanthin and lutein have antioxidant properties which help in preventing cancer, heart diseases, stroke and DNA degeneration.

Weight Loss

The main reason you are here is your weight. So let's get to the main point. Leafy green vegetables don't have fat burning properties as many people believe but they do help you in losing weight. A study conducted on overweight women with regard to the consumption of green plant membranes for three months found that eating parts of green plants that contained chlorophyll "results in significant weight reduction, and reduction in blood cholesterol together with a decreased urge for palatable food". This is the foundation of 10 day green smoothie cleanse and you will see some change in those stubborn numbers on the scale.

Other benefits include better sleep and improved energy levels.

Being healthy and energetic feels amazing, especially when you have suffered from major or minor health issues. Keep in mind that your fitness depends on good diet and lifestyle. You can achieve all that if you prepare yourself for making good changes in your life.

◆ ◆ ◆

CHAPTER 2

Getting Started

Before you start, you should know that it is one of the hardest challenges you will be accepting. If you know about the struggles you will be facing beforehand, you will stick to it with all your strength. Will-power plays a major role in getting you through anything you face. BUT it will be worth it once you complete this 10 day cleanse. You will get to know your strengths and weaknesses in a new light. AND you will see good changes in your body and mind. You will also develop patience, stamina and perseverance. These are the qualities you need to resist all the delicious but harmful foods. This detox plan is not simply about physical changes, it is more about changing the way you think about your lifestyle. Once, that is achieved, you will experience real victory. Let's make some meaningful changes in our lives!

The first 3 days will be the hardest as your body is used to whole foods and lots of calories every day. Now, you will get food in the form of green smoothies. You will naturally crave more food and it will be an uneasy feeling but as it is the time of adjustment, let yourself adjust to the new changes. Don't keep yourself hungry and snack on apples, cucumbers, carrots and any crunchy vegetables you like. This will keep your metabolism active and help you lose weight easily. When your body will slowly get used to the nutritious green smoothies, you will like drinking your smoothies and eating the allowed snacks.

As most of the food is raw: blended leafy greens, fruits, vegetables, unsalted nuts and seeds, your stomach get to relax a bit. When it doesn't get the huge amounts of all kinds of food, it works better and your body will get some time to heal and repair itself. That is the time when the body starts to focus on cleansing. Don't expect a lot of changes in this time period. You will notice the changes after this initial phase.

What SHOULD Go in the Green Smoothies?

Green smoothies are one of the easiest things you can make. Take a look at the list below of what you should be adding to your smoothies:

- Raw ingredients: leafy green vegetables, water and fruits

- Dark green leafy veggies: arugula, collard greens, bok choy, kale, mustard greens, spinach, parsley, spring greens etc.

- Fruits include apples, lemons, mangos, grapes, pears, avocado, berries, strawberries, oranges. You can go for other fruits according to the recipes. Just go easy on them and do ask your doctor if you are a diabetic.

- Almond milk is rich in protein and will make your smoothies creamy and delicious.

- Use purified water.

Stay away from Absorb all the information before you make your first smoothie. It is important to stay away from certain foods. Let's take a look at them:

- Starchy vegetables are a no-no for your smoothies during your 10 day cleanse. Carrots, potatoes, beets, or vegetables other than leafy greens should not go into your smoothies because they will cause gas and bloating.

- Refined sugar, processed foods, white bread, pasta, donuts and sugary deserts contribute to weight gain.

- Meat and dairy

- Caffeinated beverages like tea and coffee

- Sodas

- Alcohol

- Fried Foods

Don't Worry about the Cost!

While going through the shopping lists given below you might be concerned that you will have to spend a lot of money for this cleanse. It's not very expensive as you have to make all your smoothies at home. A vegetable smoothie at a juice bar will be around $7 but the same smoothie made at home will only cost you $3 on average. Unlike some popular smoothie diets and cleanses, this one doesn't need expensive protein powders and products. Get fresh ingredients from your local farmers market if you can. This will be cost effective and you will get the best produce. You can freeze the fruit so it doesn't go bad.

Grocery Shopping

The next important thing is buying everything you need. You will need these items for the **first 5 days**:

- ➢ 3 green apples
- ➢ 3 lemons
- ➢ 1 bunch kale
- ➢ Spinach – 20 ounces
- ➢ 1 bunch mint
- ➢ 1 bunch parsley
- ➢ 1 broccoli
- ➢ Romaine
- ➢ 4 stalks celery
- ➢ 1 mango
- ➢ 1 banana
- ➢ 2 oranges/5 ounces orange juice
- ➢ 2 pears
- ➢ 1 bunch grapes
- ➢ 1 avocado
- ➢ Mixed frozen berries – 20 ounces
- ➢ Frozen strawberries – 10 ounces
- ➢ Cucumbers as needed for smoothies and eating
- ➢ 10 ounces of coconut water (optional)
- ➢ A bag of salad greens
- ➢ Green tea
- ➢ Chia seeds – 1 bag
- ➢ For snacks: celery, cucumbers, apples, carrots or vegetables and fruits of your choice

There is one more list for the **next 5 days**:

- ➢ 2 oranges

- ➤ Strawberries – 10 ounces
- ➤ Spinach – 20 ounces
- ➤ Almond milk – 2 liters (optional)
- ➤ 1 pineapple
- ➤ 1 mango
- ➤ 1 pear
- ➤ Cucumbers as needed
- ➤ Flaxseed – 1 bag
- ➤ Blueberries – 20 ounces
- ➤ 2 Bananas
- ➤ Honey
- ➤ Chia seeds – 1 bag
- ➤ Fruits and veggies for snacking
- ➤ Unsalted nuts
- ➤ Green or Herbal tea of your choice

Measurements and 'Before' Picture

As with any diet and exercise regimen, you should take a 'before' picture to see the changes in your body and face. Take measurements of your waist, hips and thighs so that you can compare the difference after completing this 10 day cleanse. This is a helpful way of looking at the benefits and changes you will notice after this detox plan.

Tips for the First Day

After waking up, mentally prepare yourself for the challenge ahead. Don't worry and relax! You've got this! Think about how your health will improve in such a short period of time. You will be kicking off some of the eating habits that aren't good for you. Drink water and make herbal tea before you make your first smoothie.

IMPORTANT TIP: If you go to work early, prepare your smoothie and snacks at night so you can easily get ready for work. Pack everything with you so that it's easier to stick with the plan.

Drink lots of water because the basis of this 10 day green smoothie cleanse is to **stay hydrated.**

Tips for Achieving your Goal

Now is the time for some additional tips that will help you a lot in this 10 day green smoothie cleanse.

1. **Motivational Calendar:** Set up a motivational calendar and mark off each day and give yourself little leisure time treats like visit to the salon or movie night with your friends. This will keep you pumped up throughout this 10 day challenge.

2. **Blender:** You need a good high speed blender to make your smoothies. A large blender like Blendtec, Vitamix or any other that can hold 2 liters of smoothie is a good option. If you have a smaller blender, divide the ingredients and make half of the quantity mentioned at a time.

3. **Drink slowly** and try not to gulp it down when you are in a hurry. This is important for better digestion.

4. **Cut off the Stems:** The stems of green veggies change the taste of smoothies, so make sure to cut off the stems and put only the leaves or the main part.

5. **Add a Variety of Greens:** It's better to use a variety of greens in your smoothies. For example, you can buy spinach and kale for your smoothies one week and the next week you can go for parsley and collard greens. This way you will not be over consuming a particular vegetable.

6. **Frozen Fruits:** You can also buy frozen fruit instead of the fresh fruit. If you buy fresh fruit, freeze it so it won't go bad. However, you can also use fresh fruits in your smoothies. Also note that you don't need to freeze apples.

7. **Cool Smoothies:** Cool smoothies taste better and stay fresh for longer periods of time. Add ice if you are using fresh fruit or use frozen fruits to make cool smoothies. Keep them refrigerated and freshen up after every 4 hours with a cool glass of smoothie. Enjoy your smoothies!

8. **Make them Tasty:** As you will be drinking loads of smoothies in these 10 days, make them taste good. Sweeten them by adding the herbal sweetener called Stevia. You can add more fruit or even use a little honey in your smoothies. Add more ice or water to make them thinner. If your smoothies taste good, you will be able to complete the green smoothie cleanse with better spirits.

9. **Add Almond Milk:** Almond milk adds a creamy richness to smoothies. It's high in protein which will help in boosting your metabolism. It's optional but if you add almond milk instead of water, your smoothie will taste better and it will also add to the nutritional value of your smoothie.

10. **Herbal Tea:** Drinking herbal tea is a great way to start your morning as it has many health benefits. One of those benefits include improved metabolism, burning fat and weight loss. Herbal tea also helps in the detoxification process and managing hunger. Some of the best herbal teas you should consider are peppermint, ginseng, ginger, lemon grass and green tea. It can also help you in quitting caffeine addiction.

11. **For Diabetics:** Managing diabetes is no joke and you should never take any risk when it comes to diet. So, it's very important that you take your doctor's permission before you go along with this detox. All smoothies contain fruits, so you can switch high sugar fruits with moderate or low sugar ones. Low sugar fruits include lemon, grapefruit, and all berries. Moderate sugar fruits are pomegranate, orange, plums, peaches, apples and pears. Try not to use too many high sugar fruits like mangos, dates, grapes, pineapple, banana and melons. If your doctor gives you the GREEN SIGNAL, regularly check your blood glucose levels three times a day. If YOU can do this, then anyone can!

12. **Don't Stay Hungry:** Keep in mind that it's not a starvation diet and you are free to snack on raw fruits and vegetables like apples, celery, cucumbers and other crunchy vegetables. Consider eating high protein snacks for more energy. These include hard boiled eggs, unsweetened peanut butter and Greek yoghurt. Go for a handful of unsalted nuts. Be creative and make your snacks attractive. Combine different snack ingredients and create a variety of dishes out of them. Just keep one thing in mind, if you snack more than you need to, it will slow down your progress and you might not lose 10 pounds in 10 days.

13. **Don't Overdo the Fruits:** Fruits are good and they make the smoothies tasty but if you put too much fruit in your smoothie, it will cause spikes in your blood glucose levels. You will also experience headaches and feel very uncomfortable. Go for different fruits and put small quantity of fruits in your smoothies.

14. **Start on your Day Off:** If you work or you are a student, I would suggest you to start the detox over the weekend or when you have a day off. Doing it in spring break is also a good idea because you will experience detox symptoms. You will feel sick or tired, so you need to rest a bit during your detox. This will help you to feel better.

Marlene Adelmann says something that fits right here. "When you truly understand that your food choices are powerful and life affirming, you can exercise control and restraint without deprivation". Such powerful words and how precisely they sum up the main goal of your 10 day green smoothie cleanse!

CHAPTER 3

Detox Symptoms

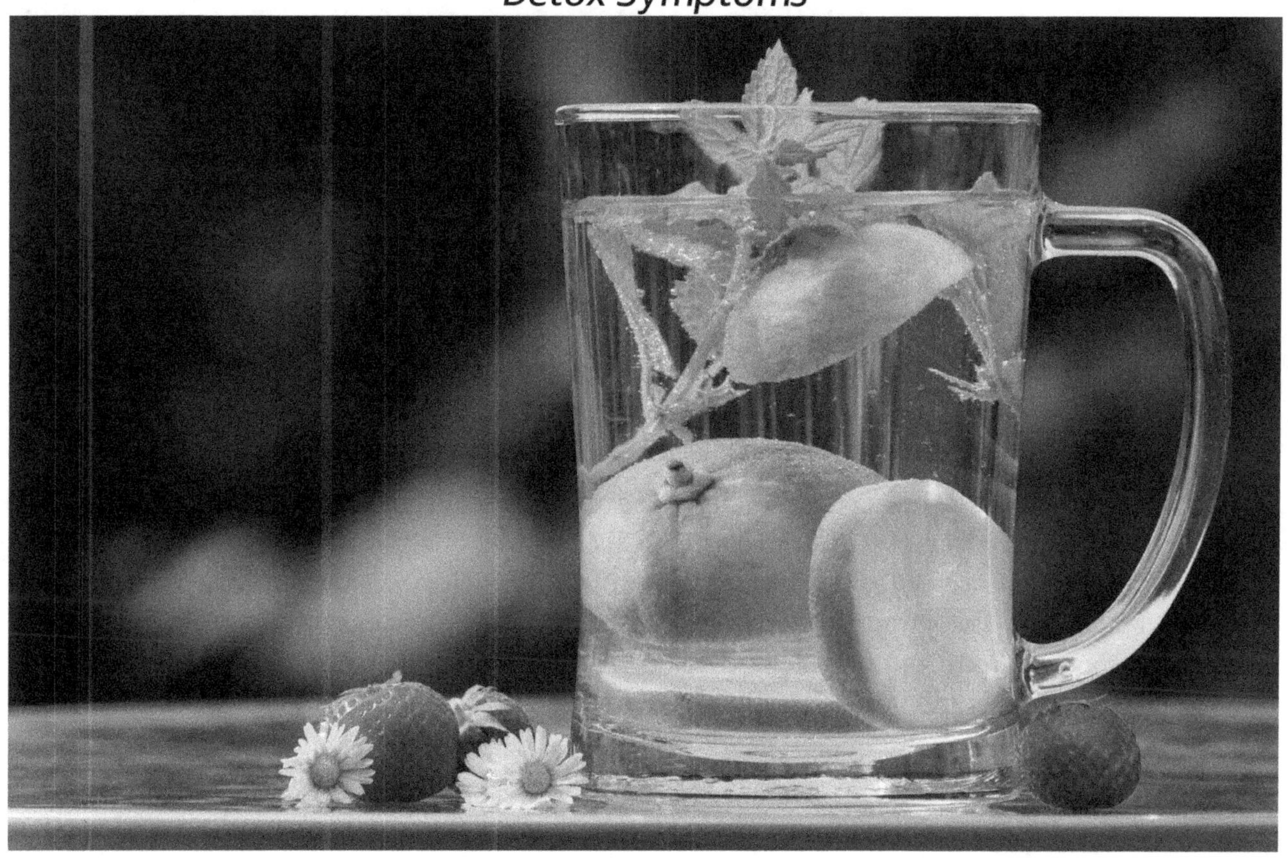

Be prepared for the next big challenge of your green smoothie cleanse and that is the detox symptoms. But don't worry because they are going to vanish after three or four days. These symptoms are unpleasant but don't think about them as something harmful. When you experience detox symptoms, it means that your body is getting rid of the toxins.

Many people argue that many vital organs like liver, kidneys and skin get rid of the toxins in our bodies and act as filters. That is true but if you look at the abundance of toxics in our environment and food, they are too much to handle for us. It affects the efficiency of the natural filters of our body and we get sick because of the toxins piling up inside us. Herbicides, pesticides, plastic, food preservatives, hormones in the chicken and meat, chemicals in almost everything and impure drinking water.

That is why we get sick and suffer from ailments like allergies, weight gain, hypertension, respiratory issues, acne and other skin problems. Even if we don't get sick, we feel sluggish and have low energy levels because we don't get the proper nutrition from our diet. Due to all these reasons, it is recommended that you should go for organic fruits and vegetables in this detox.

Now, let's discuss the detox symptoms which can make you feel very bad but they are actually the indicators of your progress. Don't worry! I am going to tell you how to deal with these symptoms.

Headaches and Pains

If you drink a lot of tea or coffee, then you should expect headaches for three or four days after starting the green smoothie cleanse. It's difficult for the first timers, especially if you suffer from migraines. You can also experience joint pains or pain in any part of the body.

Don't take any pain killer because it will be counterproductive to the detox and the pain might get worse. Try massage therapy as it will improve the blood flow and will ease the tension. Massage your temples and forehead in circular motion with your fingertips for a few minutes. Massage is also good for getting relief from other physical pains. Also, try putting ice on the affected area. Cover the ice with a thin cloth or put it in a sealable plastic bag. Do this for 10-15 minutes and you will feel better.

Bowel Discomfort and Gas

The detox directly affects the digestive system. So, you'll feel discomfort in the stomach and have frequent bowel movements in the first few days. The green smoothie cleanse is comprised of high fiber smoothies and snacks and your body might not be used to so much raw food. This is usually a reaction of your body towards this sudden change in the diet and eating habits.

Besides digestive issues in the beginning, you will also pass gas as the body tries to get rid of the toxins. Apply the amazing chamomile oil to minimize this common symptom.

Keep yourself hydrated and you can also take psyllium husk by mixing it with plain yoghurt or by adding a tablespoon to a glass of water. It provides so much relief. As for all the other detox symptoms, digestive disturbance will also go away after the first 4 days.

Fatigue and Weakness

You will be tired and feel weak as the body goes through the detoxification process. Just give yourself time to rest and avoid social events for a few days. This is a temporary effect of the detox and once your body gets used to the new change, you will be energetic and happy. If you are extremely exhausted, avoid physical exertion for a few days. You can resume your exercise routine after 5 days or even after the 10 day cleanse.

Skin Rashes

When our body is fighting germs or it is getting rid of the toxins through skin, we get skin rashes and even acne sometimes. The best natural remedy without any side effects is Aloe Vera. Apply Aloe Vera to sooth your skin rashes and get rid of the acne. Drinking loads of water is highly recommended to make the rashes and pimples go away.

Flu-like Symptoms

You can also experience flu-like symptoms and feel that your body is breaking down. Herbal tea will be really helpful and take a nap to freshen up.

Mood Swings

You will be irritable and moody as you have to avoid many of your favorite foods. Divert your attention from eating and do something useful. Keep yourself busy and you will be less cranky.

Cravings

When the detox starts, you naturally crave the food you used to eat like sugar, dairy, coffee and meat. As you reduce your solid food intake and drink smoothies most of the time, you will desire solid food more. This will only last for the first four or five days. After that, the cravings will go away but you can get bored from your new routine. As for the hunger part, this green smoothie cleanse focuses on nourishment instead of starvation. So, you will not be hungry most of the time except when you wake up in the morning with empty stomach.

To deal with your hunger and cravings, take in as much water as you can and keep drinking a glass of smoothie after every 3-4 hours. Don't skip your snacks and make them as palatable as you like within the prescribed limits. When you will be fuller, you will not desire other foods and coffee.

Be strong during the detox phase! You will need all your strength and will power to get through these 10 important days of your life. Just remember that these symptoms will last for only a few days. However, if they are too strong, you can follow these guidelines:

1. Put more fruit and less vegetables in your smoothies in the beginning. After that, keep on reducing the amount of fruit and put more vegetables when you get used to drinking smoothies and your detox symptoms go away.

2. For Day One, drink one glass of smoothie for breakfast and have a healthy salad or filling snack for lunch and dinner.

3. Go for 2 glasses of smoothie for Day Two i.e. for breakfast and lunch. Eat a healthy snack at night.

4. Try drinking your smoothie for the whole day on Day Three. If you are not fully ready for that, take a snack like a big salad for one meal.

Hopefully, you will feel better after the initial detox phase. Here is another beautiful quote for you, "If you are tired of starting over, stop giving up". Buckle up and get ready for this thrilling and life-changing ride!

◆ ◆ ◆

CHAPTER 4

10 Daily Smoothie Recipes

These core smoothie recipes for your 10 day green smoothie cleanse are designed to detox your body, lose weight and boost energy. The shopping lists provided contain all the ingredients you need to make these delicious and healthy smoothies. You can be creative if you want to AFTER the detox. It's better to stick with these recipes as much as you can to lose 10 pounds in 10 days. Plus, they taste great to keep you motivated throughout the detox.

IMPORTANT: If you have a full-sized blender like Blendtec or Vitamix, you can easily make 2 liters of smoothie. If it's smaller, you need to divide the recipe and blend twice to make your smoothie for the whole day.

Now, let's get started!

Day 1: Green Lemonade Smoothie

Green lemonade offers many health benefits. You will be delighted to know that it not only helps you in losing weight but it also keeps your heart healthy. Apples contain compounds that delay the breakdown of LDL i.e. bad cholesterol. Lemons help in boosting the immune system and reducing weight. Greens such as spinach, mint, kale, collard, coriander, chard etc. are also very beneficial for your health, especially spinach because it is rich in potassium, iron, fiber, lutein and folate.

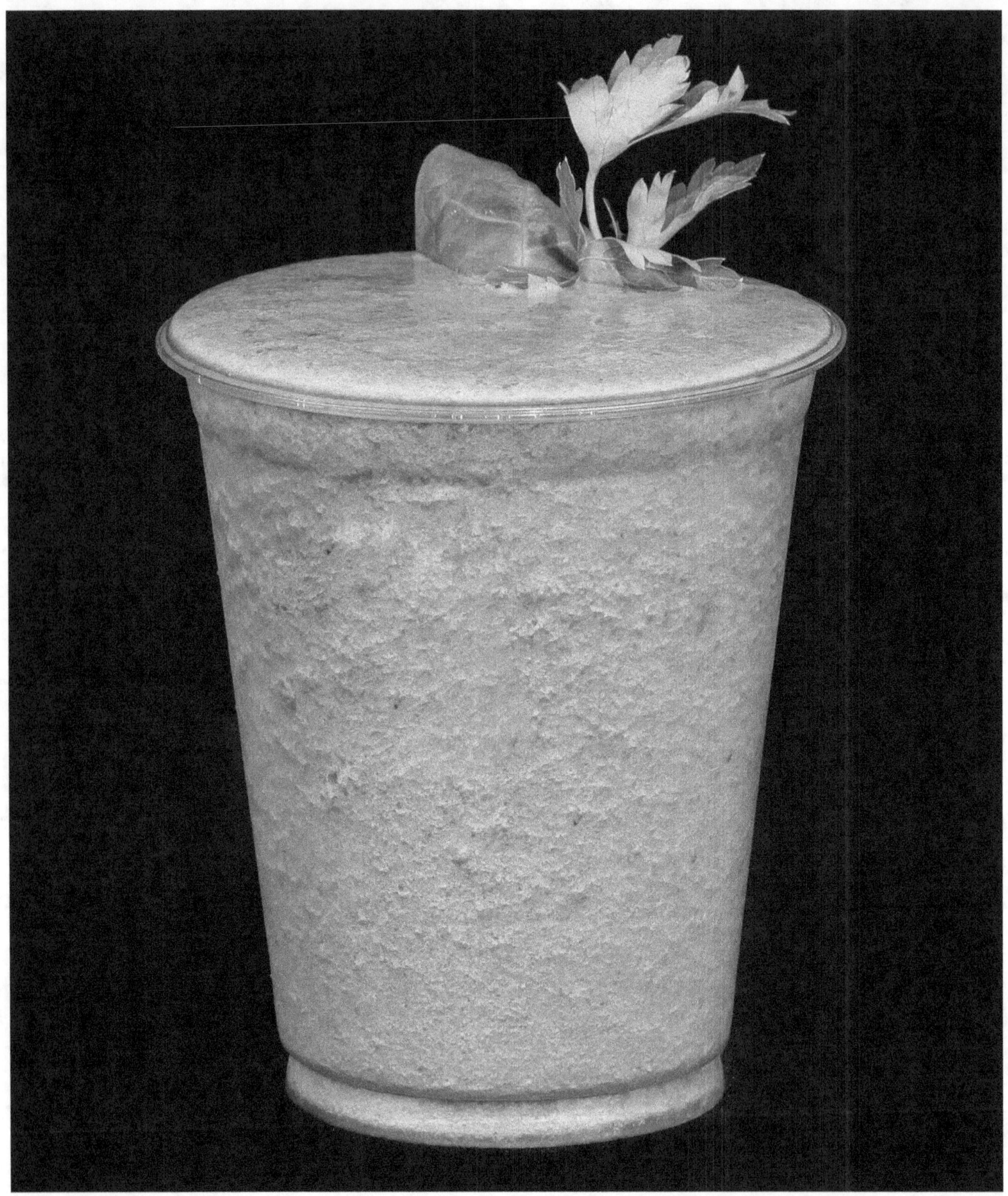

Ingredients:

1) A peeled lemon
2) 2 green apples
3) 2 handfuls spinach or any other green mentioned above

Blend and drink this amazing weight loss smoothie.

Day 2: Green Detox Smoothie

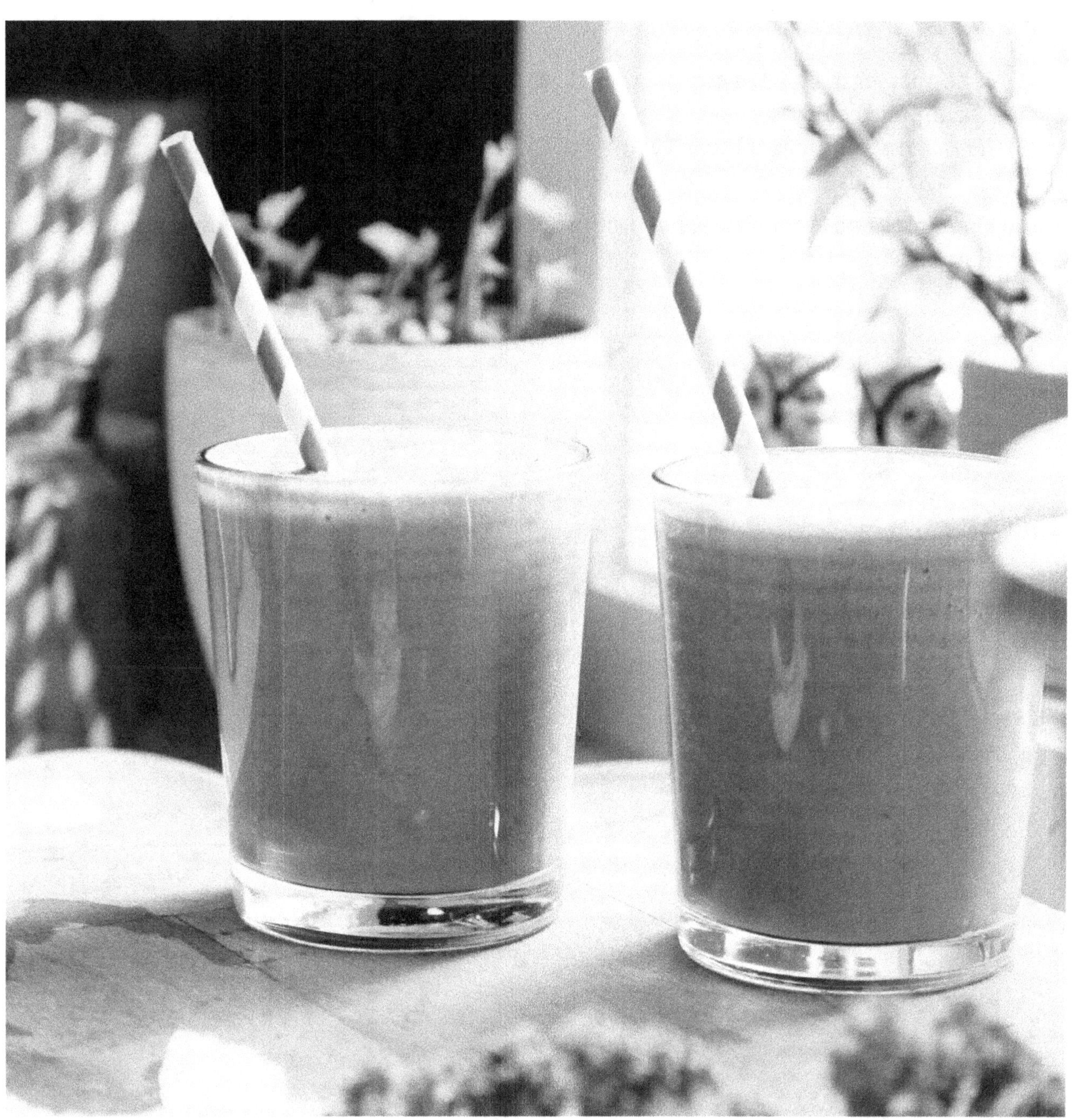

This smoothie contains a variety of greens. So, it's rich in iron and anti-oxidants. Plus, the high fiber content of this smoothie will help with constipation and weight loss.

Ingredients:

1) Fresh chopped mint – 1/4 cup
2) Chopped kale leaves – 1/4 cup
3) Chopped parsley – 1/4 cup
4) 2 chopped celery
5) Fresh orange juice – 1 cup
6) Mango cubes – 1 cup

Blend them nice and smooth and keep sipping this healthy and delicious green smoothie the entire day.

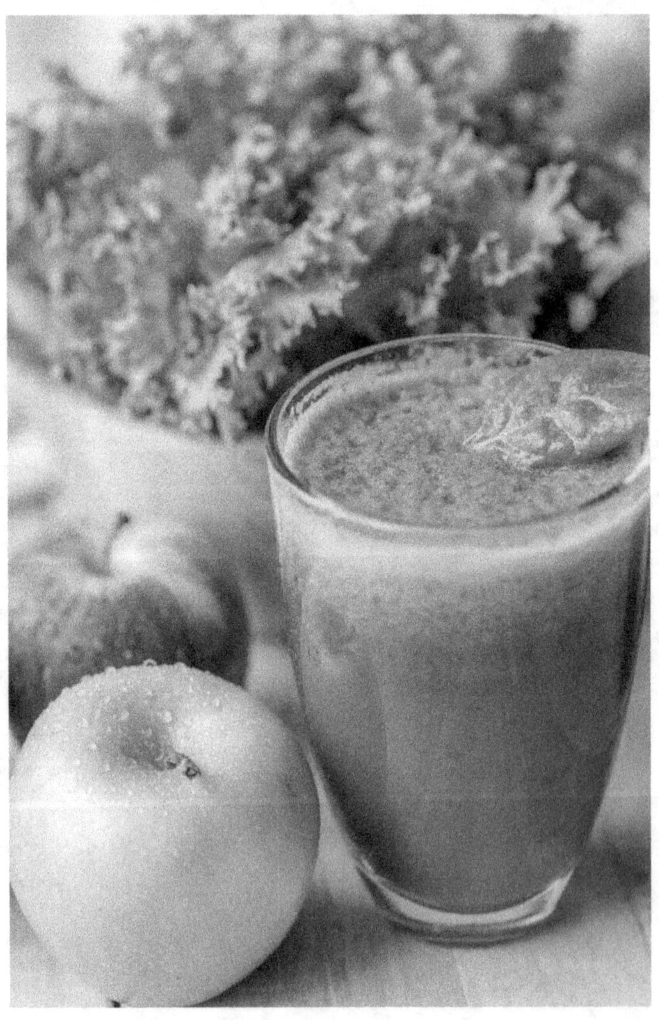

Day 3: Kale and Ginger Smoothie

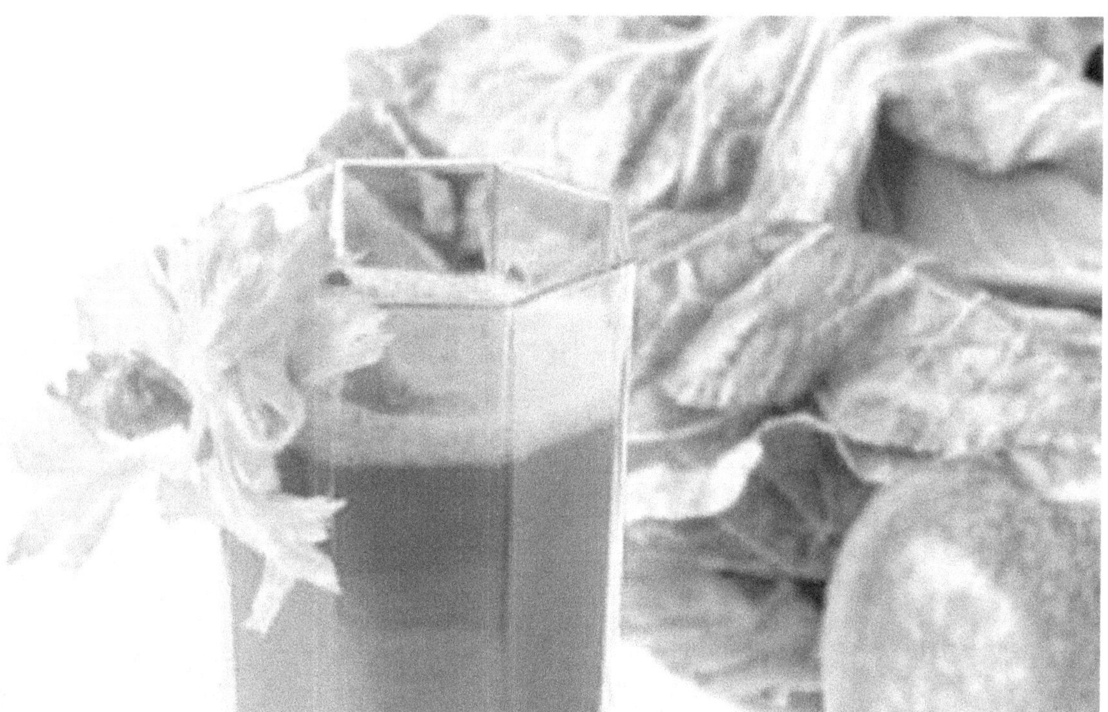

Kale and ginger is a superb combination. Kale has so much to offer for your health and ginger aids in digestion. Let's give it a go for our third day!

Ingredients:

1) Kale – 1 cup
2) Ginger – half inch
3) 1/4 avocado
4) Half cucumber
5) Half lemon
6) Coconut water – 1/2 cup
7) Water

Put everything in a blender, give it a whirl and you have a tasty and healthy green smoothie.

Day 4: Fresh Cucumber Smoothie

Making cucumber the base of your smoothie is a wise choice. It makes a good combination with leafy greens and keeps you hydrated throughout the day.

Ingredients:

1) 1 Cucumber
2) A fistful of kale
3) A fistful of romaine
4) 2 stalks of celery
5) 1 green apple
6) Half peeled lemon

Make a nice smoothie and freshen up each time you drink.

Day 5: Scrumptious Grape Smoothie

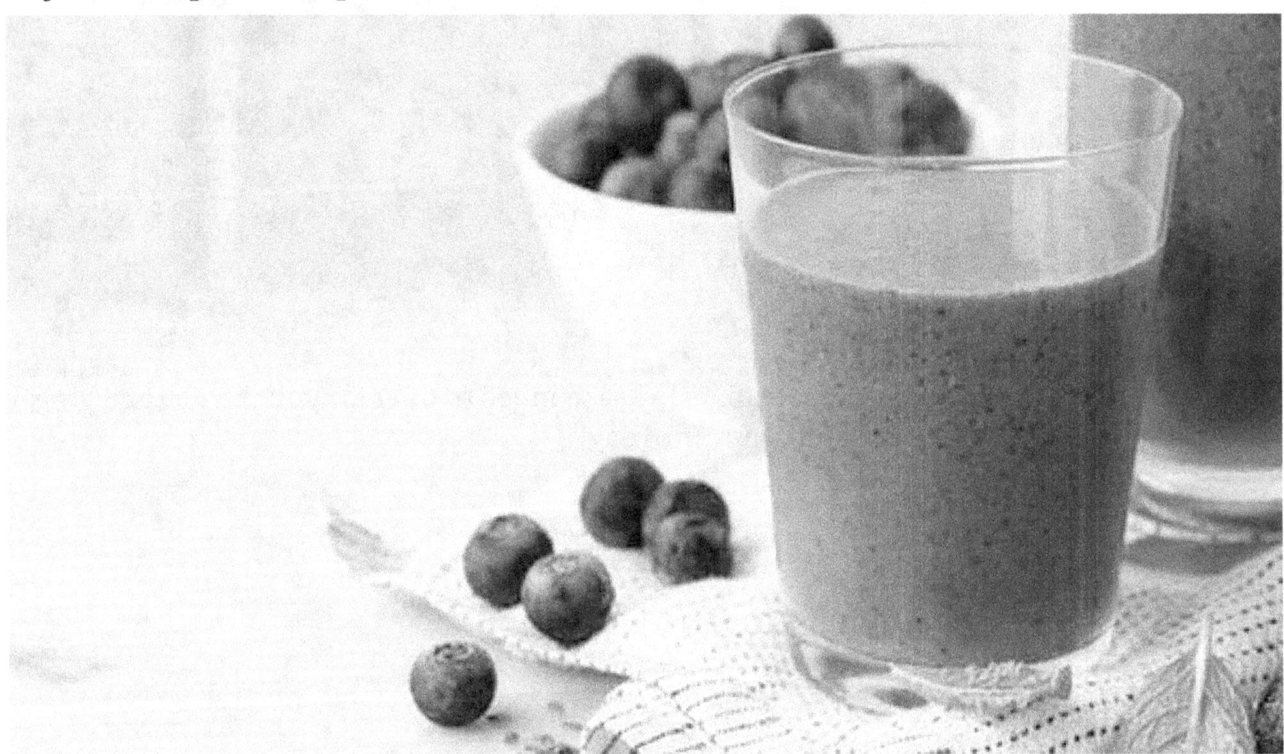

Grapes are not just mouth-watering, they pack so much energy when combined with kale and spinach. Adding other fruits like banana, orange and pear gives it a nice fruity flavor. You will enjoy it on the fifth day of detox.

Ingredients:

1) Green grapes – 1 cup
2) Spinach – 1 cup
3) Kale – 1 cup
4) A pear with its seeds, core and stem removed
5) 1 banana
6) 1 orange
7) Chia seeds – 1 tsp
8) ½ cup of water
9) Ice – 1/2 cup

Put all the ingredients in your blender and blend at slow speed for about 20 seconds. Then move to medium and high speed within the next 60 seconds. In less than 2 minutes, you'll have yourself a wonderful green smoothie.

Day 6: Amazing Spinach and Strawberry Smoothie

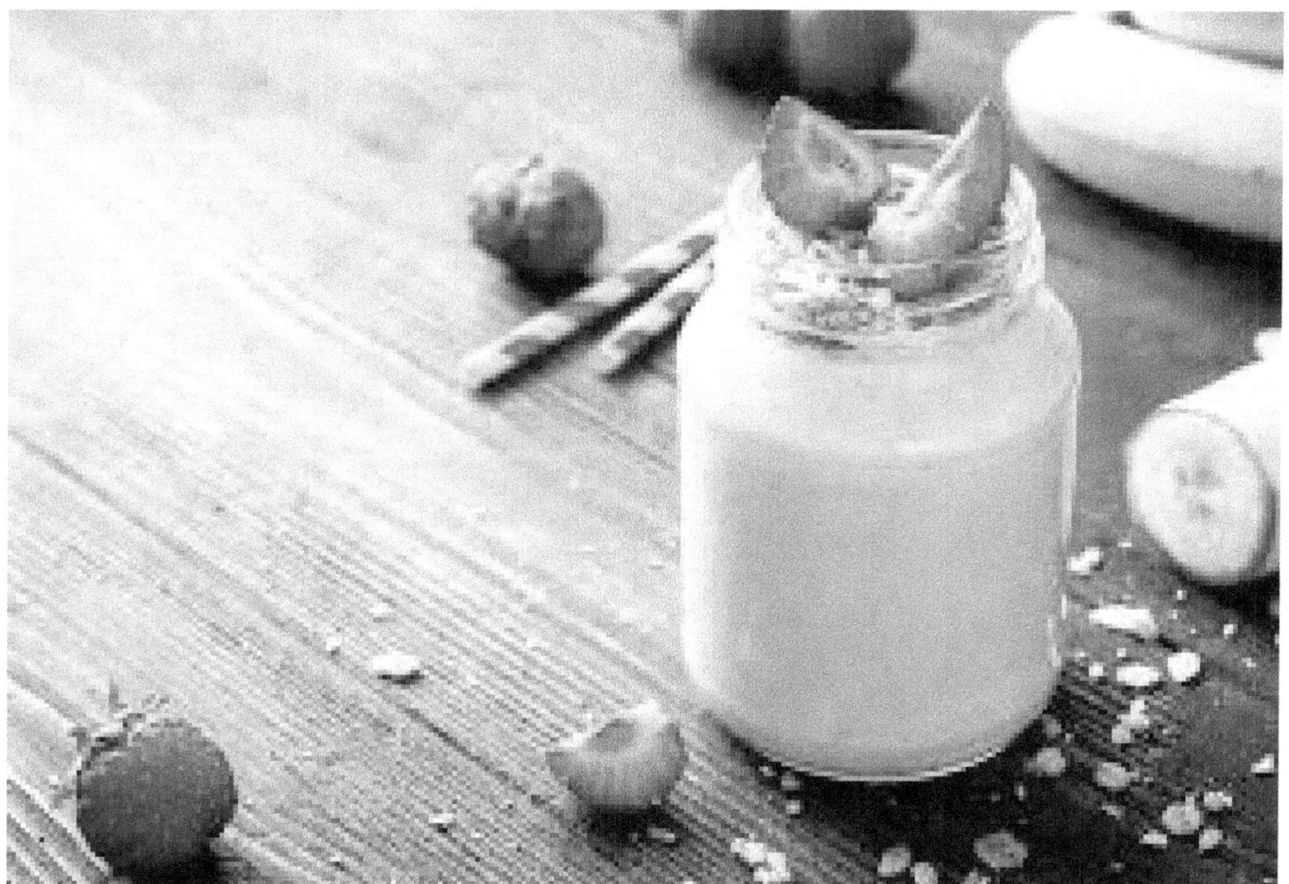

Add some twist in this classic spinach smoothie by adding strawberries and orange. Also, boost your metabolism by adding almond milk.

Ingredients:
1) Raw Spinach – 1 cup
2) Strawberries – 1/3 cup
3) 1 orange
4) Almond milk – 1 cup

Blend everything to a nice and smooth consistency.

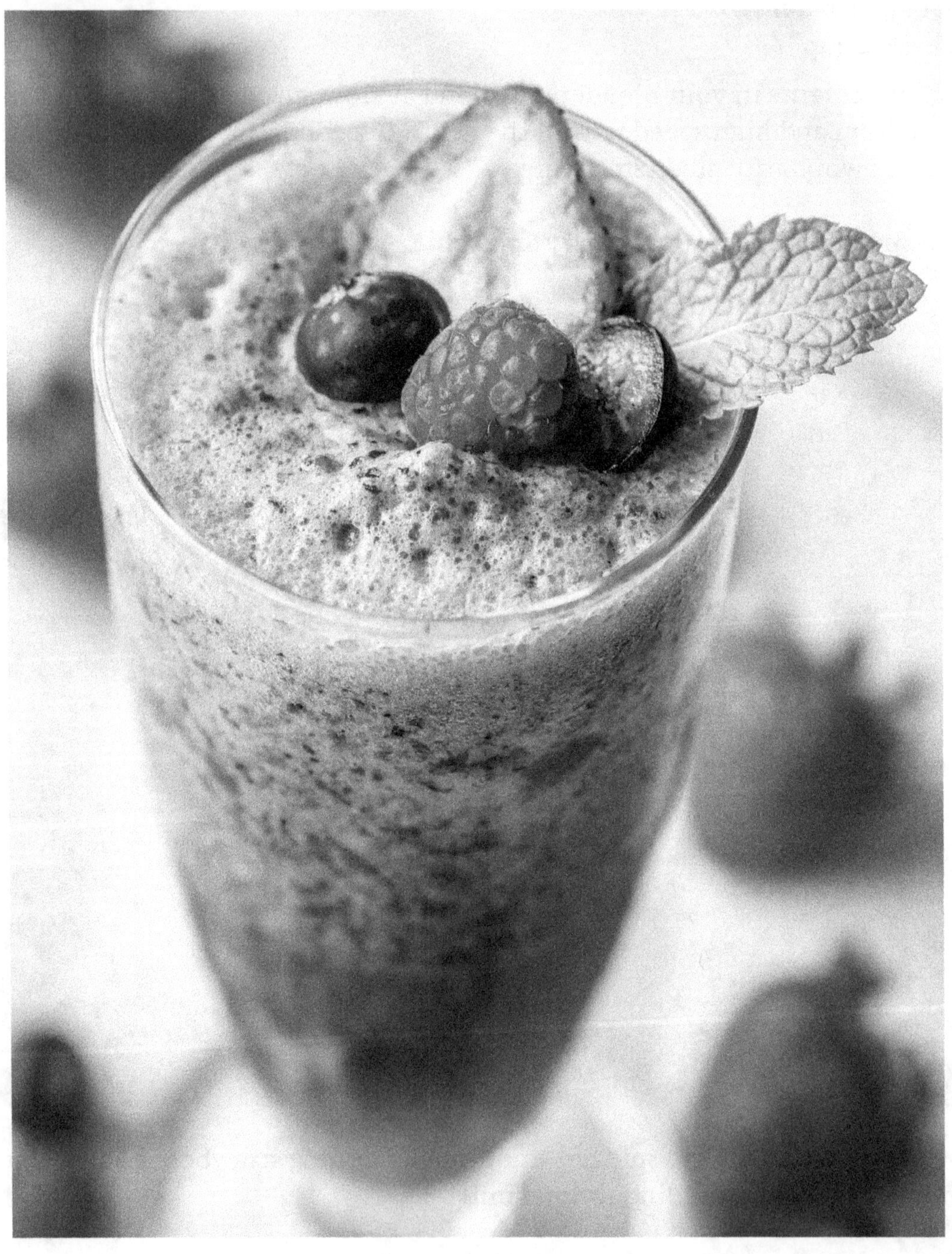

Day 7: Spinach and Kale Smoothie

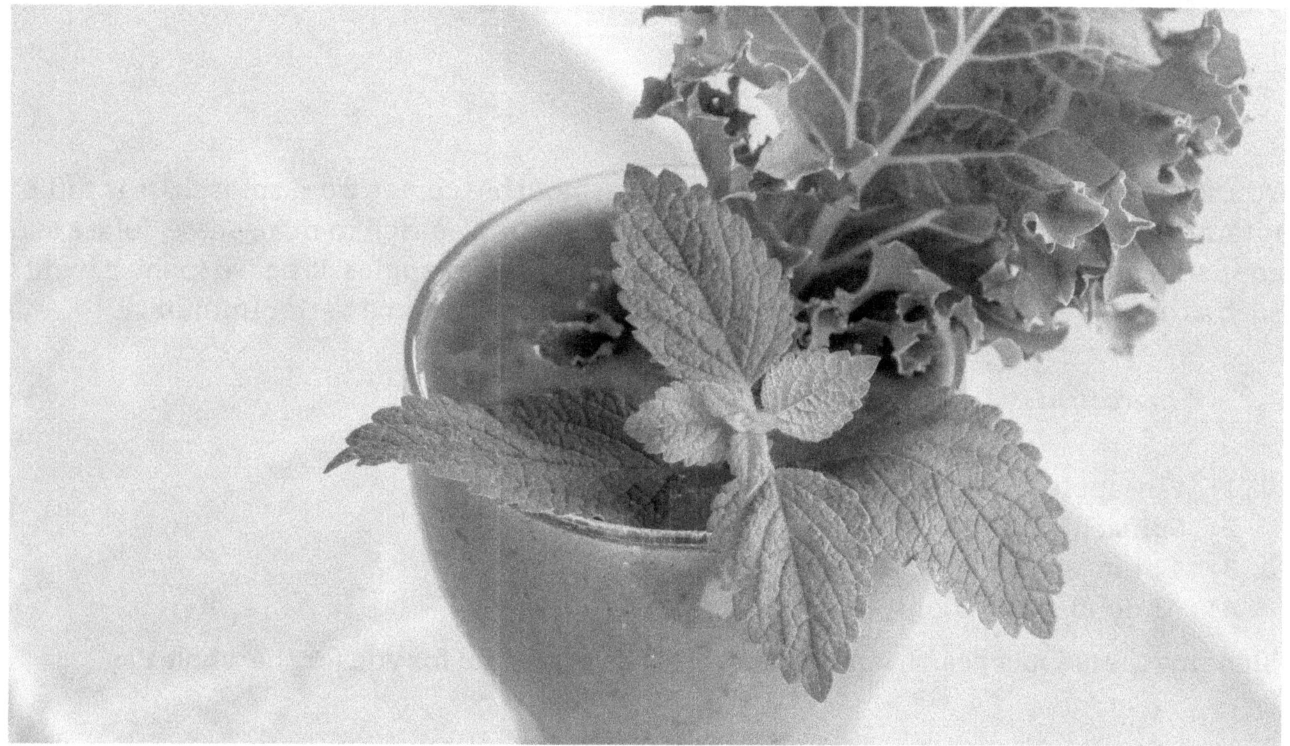

The goal of drinking these smoothies is not just losing weight. You need to look fresh and let me tell you the secret behind gorgeous skin – kale! It's full of carotenoids which gives your skin a healthy touch and makes it glow. Not only that, it also protects your skin from wrinkles. Drinking this smoothie is a perfect way to make your skin glow while you lose weight. Adding fruits like banana, grapes, pear and orange enhance the flavor and make you feel amazing throughout the day.

Ingredients:

1) Spinach – 1cup
2) Kale – 1 cup
3) Green grapes – 1cup
4) 1 orange
5) 1 pear
6) 1 banana
7) Chia seeds – 1 tsp

8) Water – half cup
9) Ice – 1/2 cup

Chop kale, spinach and pear. Blend them first and then add the rest of the ingredients and blend on high speed. Enjoy your smoothie!

Day 8: Pineapple Smoothie

You see the bright green color of this pineapple smoothie comes from spinach. It is full of vitamin C because of pineapple and orange. Pineapple is also rich in manganese, folate and copper. A plant compound called bromelain is found in pineapples. It has so many benefits such as improved digestion, fighting cancer, healing properties and better immunity.

Ingredients:

1) Pineapple – 1/4 cup
2) Spinach – 1 cup
3) 1 orange
4) Almond milk – 1 cup

Blending these super healthy ingredients will be very useful for you for the whole day.

Day 9: Sweet Mango Cucumber Smoothie

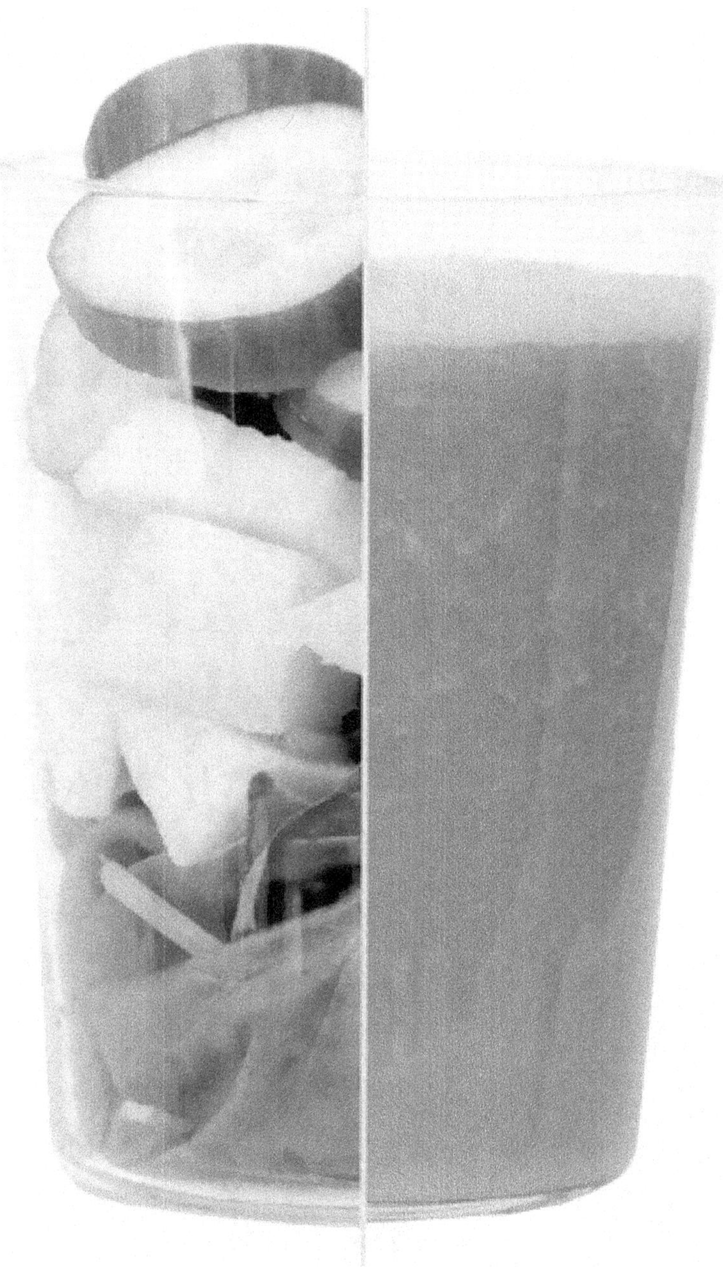

Here you have a very delicious mango cucumber smoothie. Thanks to the mangoes, you've got great flavor and lots of vitamins! Ingredients:

1) *Mangoes – 1/4 cup*

2) Chopped Cucumber – 1 cup
3) 1 orange

4) Flaxseed – 1 tbsp.
5) Spinach – 1 cup

Make a smooth drink and stay fresh!

Day 10: Kale and Blueberry Smoothie

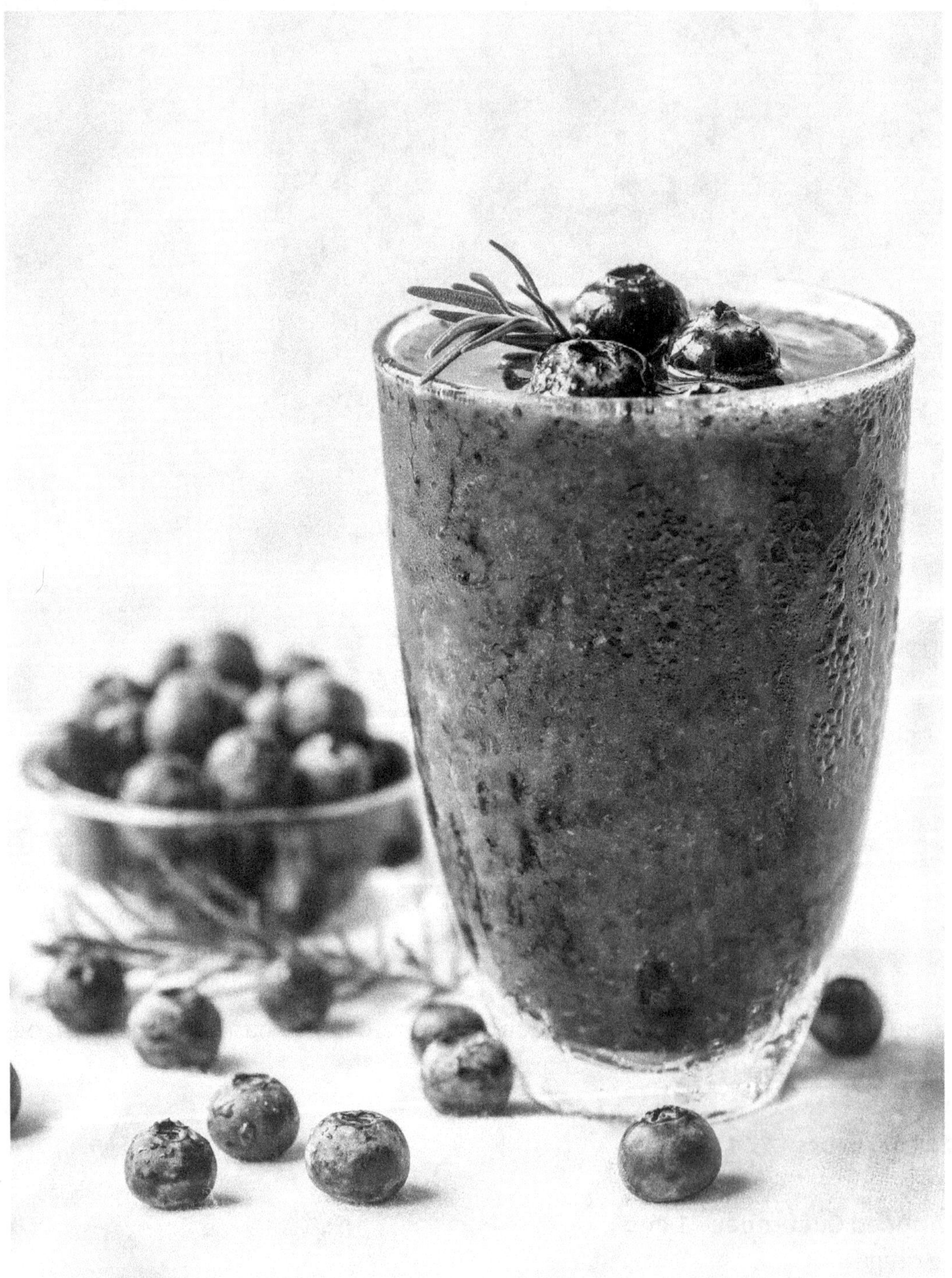

This is called hiding your greens and making it appealing for the whole family. The dark color of blueberries will hide kale and you will love the flavor. You will get antioxidants from blueberries and cherries. Kale, on the other hand, is pretty amazing because it has very few calories. Besides helping you to lose weight, it has loads of vitamin C which will boost your immunity.

Ingredients:

1) Kale – 1 cup
2) Blueberries – 1/2 cup
3) Cherries – 1/2 cup
4) Honey – 2 tsp
5) Almond milk – 1 cup

Make a creamy and tasty smoothie out of these amazing ingredients.

Best wishes for these 10 important days of your life. Try to include smoothies even after the detox in your daily routine. This will be helpful for you and your family in maintaining a healthy lifestyle. Drink these smoothies and see for yourself what a drink of green veggies and fruits can do for you. Your goal should not be to look "perfect". You will lose weight but the most important part is that you should *feel healthy*.

◆ ◆ ◆

CHAPTER 5

Snack Time

I have stressed a lot on drinking green smoothies throughout the day. But you still need to eat something light whenever you are hungry. Consider it as a safeguard against extreme hunger and cravings. Just munching on plain crunchy vegetables and eating these snacks the boring way can drive you nuts! Trust me, I tried it for two days and then the chef inside me woke up and told me to bring some twist in the boring snacks. So, I am here with some ideas for your precious snack time!

Deviled Eggs

Make deviled eggs (without the mayo) and even put any South Asian spices like chat masala or garam masala on top! Yum!

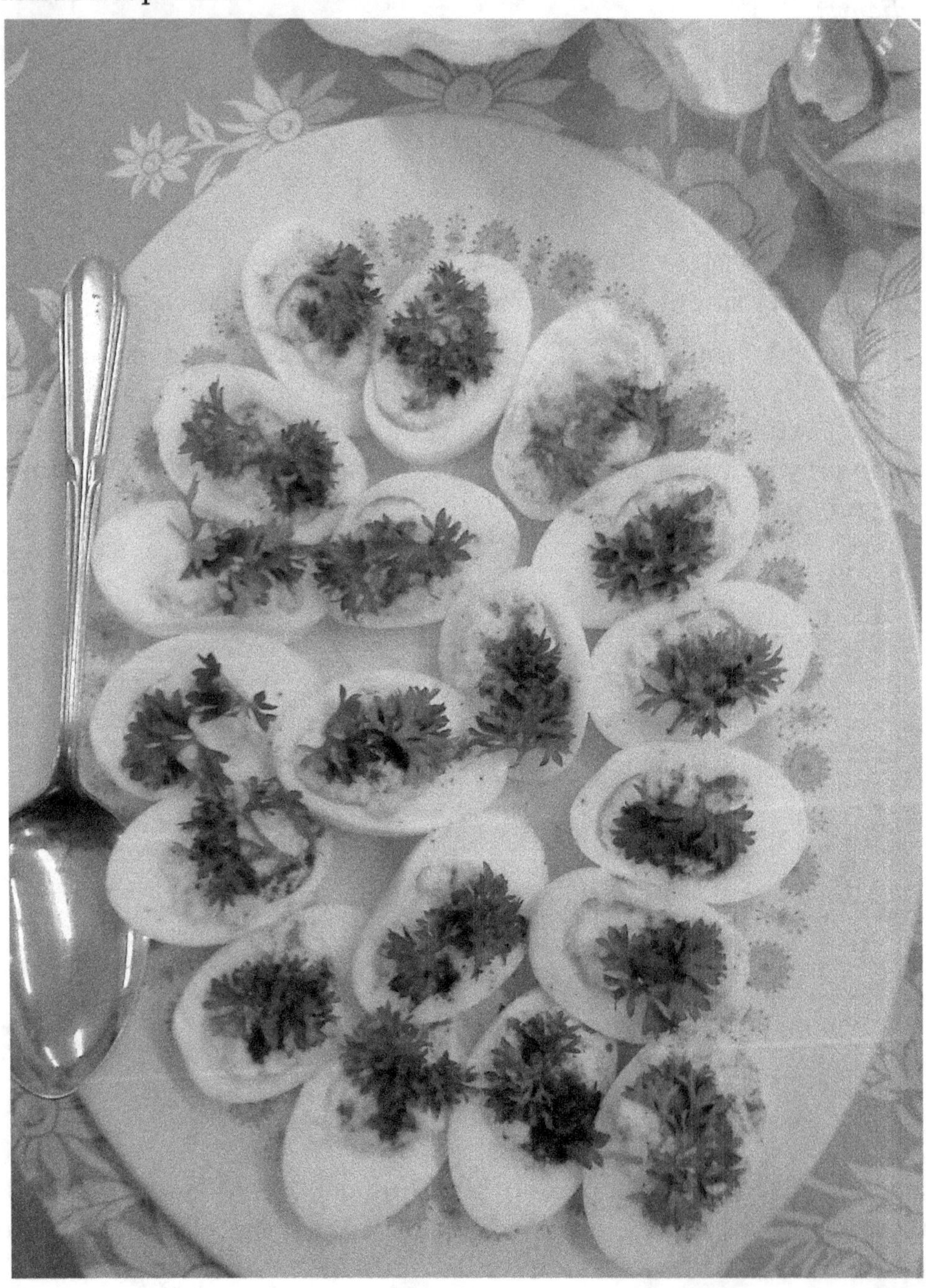

Cucumber Raita

Make cucumber raita with Greek yoghurt. Add parsley, mint, and season with a pinch of salt and chat masala.

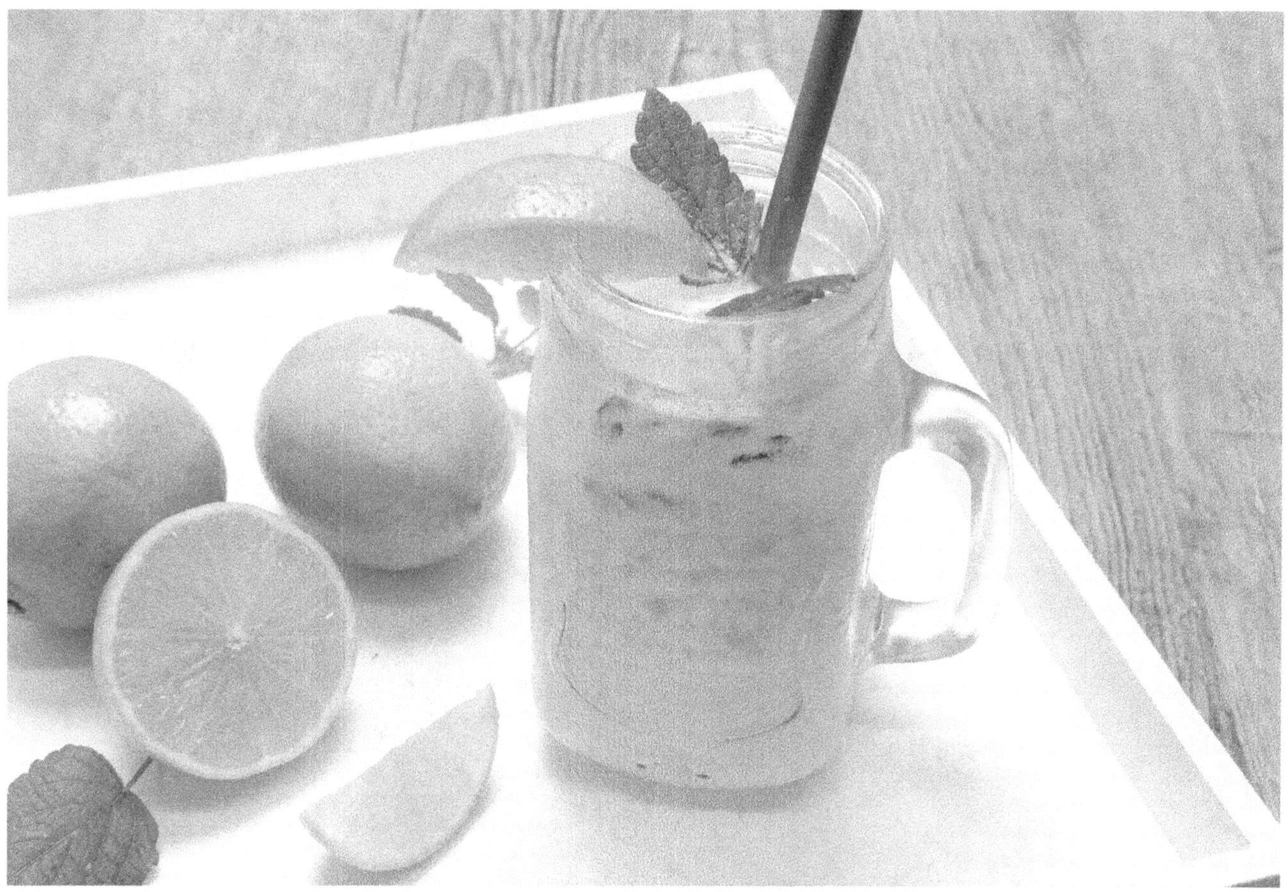

Raw Cashew Dip with Veggies

Make the cashew dip and enjoy raw veggies with this creamy and amazing dip.

Ingredients:

1) Raw cashews – 1 cup
2) Water – 3/4 cup
3) Garlic – 1 tsp
4) Apple cider vinegar – 2 tsp

5) Dill weed – 1 tsp
6) Parsley – 2 tsp
7) Chives – 1 tsp
8) Garlic powder – 1/4 tsp

Method:

- Soak cashews in water for two hours and then drain the water.
- Put in a food processor and add all ingredients.
- Blend until creamy and smooth.
- Season with salt and black pepper.

Broccoli Salad

Add any twist you like to simple salads. This broccoli salad contains apples and walnuts.

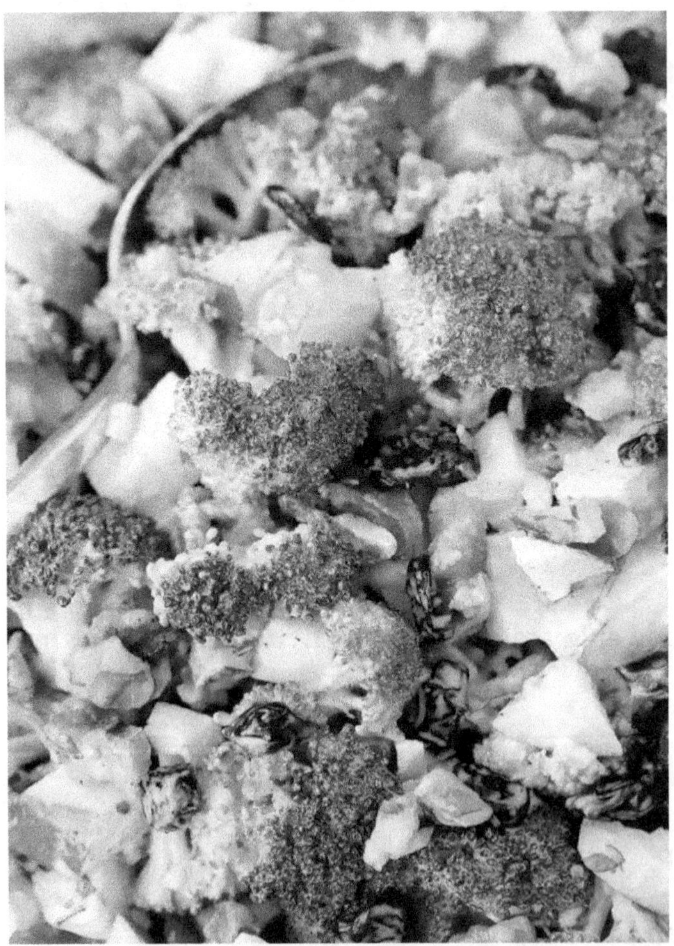

Ingredients:

1) Broccoli – 2 cups
2) 1 apple
3) Parsley – 2 tbsp.
4) Red onion – 1/2 cup
5) Cashew dip – 2 tbsp.
6) Walnuts – 1 cup

Method:

- Nicely chop broccoli, apple, parsley and red onion.
- Then add walnuts and cashew dip.
- Season with salt and black pepper.

Enjoy this hearty salad!

Peanut Butter and Apple Balls

Who says that all your snacks should be savory? You can make desserts without sugar to satisfy your sweet tooth. Just like these pretty little peanut butter and apple balls.

Ingredients:

1) Almonds – 1 cup
2) Peanut butter – 2 tbsp.
3) Grated apples – 3 tbsp.
4) Cinnamon – 1 tsp
5) Vanilla extract – 1 tsp

Method:

- Grind dry almonds to make almond flour.
- Put almond flour in a bowl and add the rest of the ingredients.
- Make balls and refrigerate for 4 hours.

Kids also love such appetizing snacks. Make some more balls if you have kids at home.

Cucumber Salad

You can make simple things taste good like this cucumber salad. Simply add sliced onions, cucumbers and the creamy cashew sauce in a bowl. Season with dill, garlic powder, salt and black pepper. Add only a quarter teaspoon of these seasonings. Add half teaspoon or more dill if you want to.

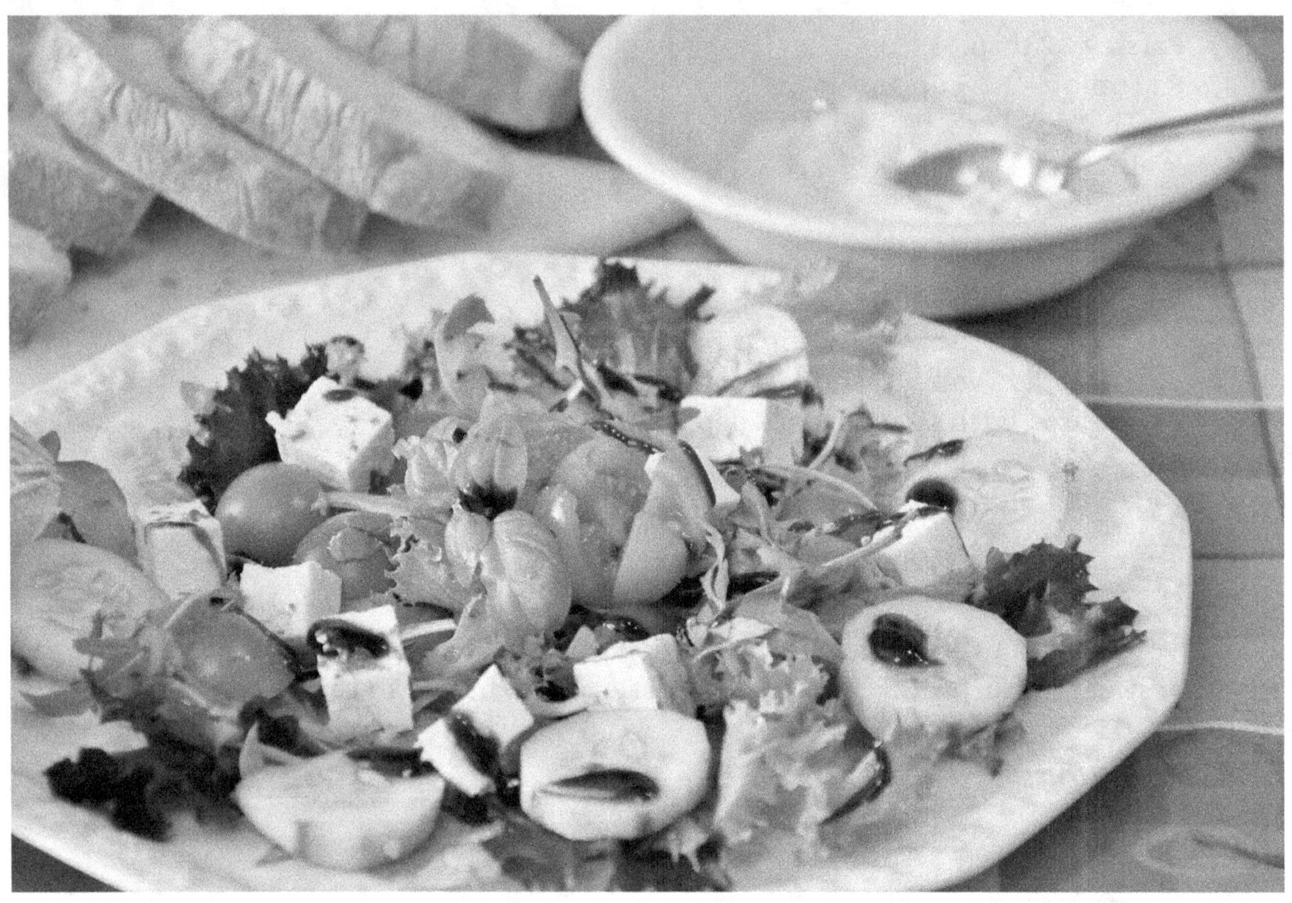

Celery Sticks Stuffed with Peanut Butter

There can be simpler options like eating your celery sticks with peanut butter. Its filling and you don't have to put extra effort in making this snack. Just stuff the sticks with peanut butter on a busy day.

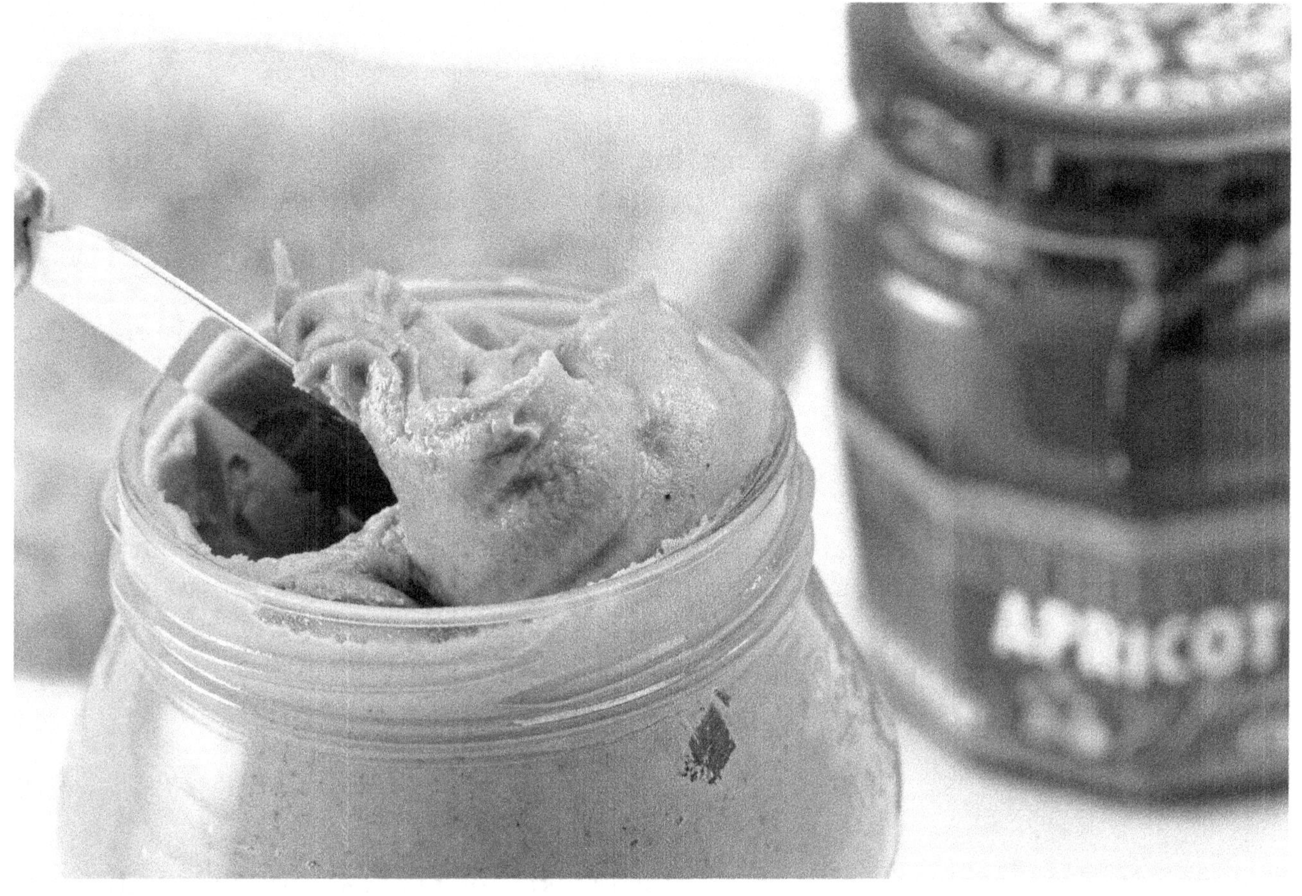

Peanut Butter and Pumpkin Dip

Now, this is called a YUMMY snack that makes you smile and fills your stomach. You can even share these recipes with health conscious friends and family members.

Ingredients:

1) Cashew dip or cream – 1/4 cup
2) Peanut butter – 1 tbsp.
3) Raw blended pumpkin – 1/4 cup
4) Pumpkin pie spice – 1/4 tsp
5) Vanilla extract – 1 tsp
6) Cinnamon – 1 tsp
7) 2 apples

Method:

- Take a bowl and mix peanut butter, blended pumpkin, pumpkin pie spice, cashew cream, cinnamon and vanilla extract.
- Slice apples and squeeze a lemon on them. You can even use celery or carrots for dipping in this tasty sauce.

You can throw a pinch of pumpkin pie spice on the apples for extra taste. Heartily enjoy this filling and delicious snack.

Snacks with Peanut Butter

Adding peanut butter to your allowed snacks is a good idea. Drizzle peanut butter over apples and crunchy veggies. Cut apples in round slices and make peanut butter sandwich. Add your own twist to each of these snacks. Make your snacks presentable with peanut butter. Sprinkle nuts over vegetable slices and drizzle a little peanut butter. But be careful in using it in small quantities as it is high in fat.

Egg Snacks

Eggs are a good source of protein as you are mostly taking plant based smoothies and snacks. Eat simple hard boiled eggs and use them in salads.

Classic No-Mayo Egg Salad

Instead of using mayo, use cashew cream or soak almonds overnight. Drain and grind them with very little water to make almond cream. It can be smooth or a slight grainy texture is also good. You will find this slight change in the recipe surprisingly pleasant.

Ingredients:
1) 2 chopped hard boiled eggs
2) A half chopped bell pepper
3) 1 chopped carrot
4) Almond cream
5) Paprika

Method:

Mix all ingredients and sprinkle paprika on top. You can use black pepper or any other spice you like instead of paprika. Make this simple and tasty egg salad to boost your energy.

Romaine Egg Salad

Eggs have this universal quality that you can combine them with so many vegetables, especially the leafy greens. Make a simple romaine salad and mix it with hard boiled eggs. You can add curry powder to enhance the taste.

TIP: Throw in other crunchy greens like zucchini, cucumber, celery and other leafy greens to make a big salad if you feel like eating something big and filling. The good thing about these veggies and eggs is that you get less calories, more fiber and more energy. They are a true blessing for people who are trying to lose weight. Eating salads like this will satiate you and you will not get hungry for a long period of time.

Veggie Hummus

Looking around for ideas in different cuisines makes you more creative. You start respecting and appreciating other cultures and diets. You might even adopt some of the healthy and delicious foods they have to offer. Hummus is usually made with chickpeas but in this detox, try making hummus with zucchini.

Ingredients:

1) Two zucchinis
2) Greek yoghurt – 1/2 cup
3) Lemon juice – 1 tbsp.
4) Olive oil – 1/3 cup
5) Cumin – 2 tsps.
6) 3 cloves of garlic

Method:

Peel and chop zucchinis. Then put everything in a food processor and make a smooth paste. Serve with crunchy raw vegetables, such as broccoli, carrots, cucumber and celery sticks.

Salads

There is so much variety in salads. You can use cucumbers in different combinations. They go well with onions, tomatoes, and Greek yogurt. You can even make a sour cucumber salad by using apple cider vinegar. Use a bunch of greens and make dressing with cashew dip or almond paste. Adding lime juice makes a perfect and fresh salad. Garnish with parsley or other herbs.

Raw Veggie Pastas

If you have a spiralizer, you can make raw veggie pastas using different allowed ingredients.

Carrot Pasta with Lime, Ginger and Peanut Sauce

Carrot pasta is a simple but exceedingly delicious and healthy pasta recipe that makes use of basic ingredients like raw carrots, cashews, peanut butter, ginger, and lime juice, etc.

Ingredients for Pasta:
1) 5 Large peeled carrots, spiraled into noodles
2) Finely sliced fresh cilantro – 2 tbsp.
3) Roasted cashews – 1/3 cup

Ingredients for Sauce:

1) Peanut Butter – 2 tbsp.
2) A pinch of cayenne pepper
3) 2 garlic cloves (diced)
4) Diced fresh ginger – 1 tbsp.
5) Lemon juice – 1 tbsp.

Method:
- Wash and peel the carrots. Make noodles using a spiralizer.
- Mix the ingredients of sauce in a bowl.
- Pour sauce on the carrots.
- Decorate with cashews and fresh cilantro.

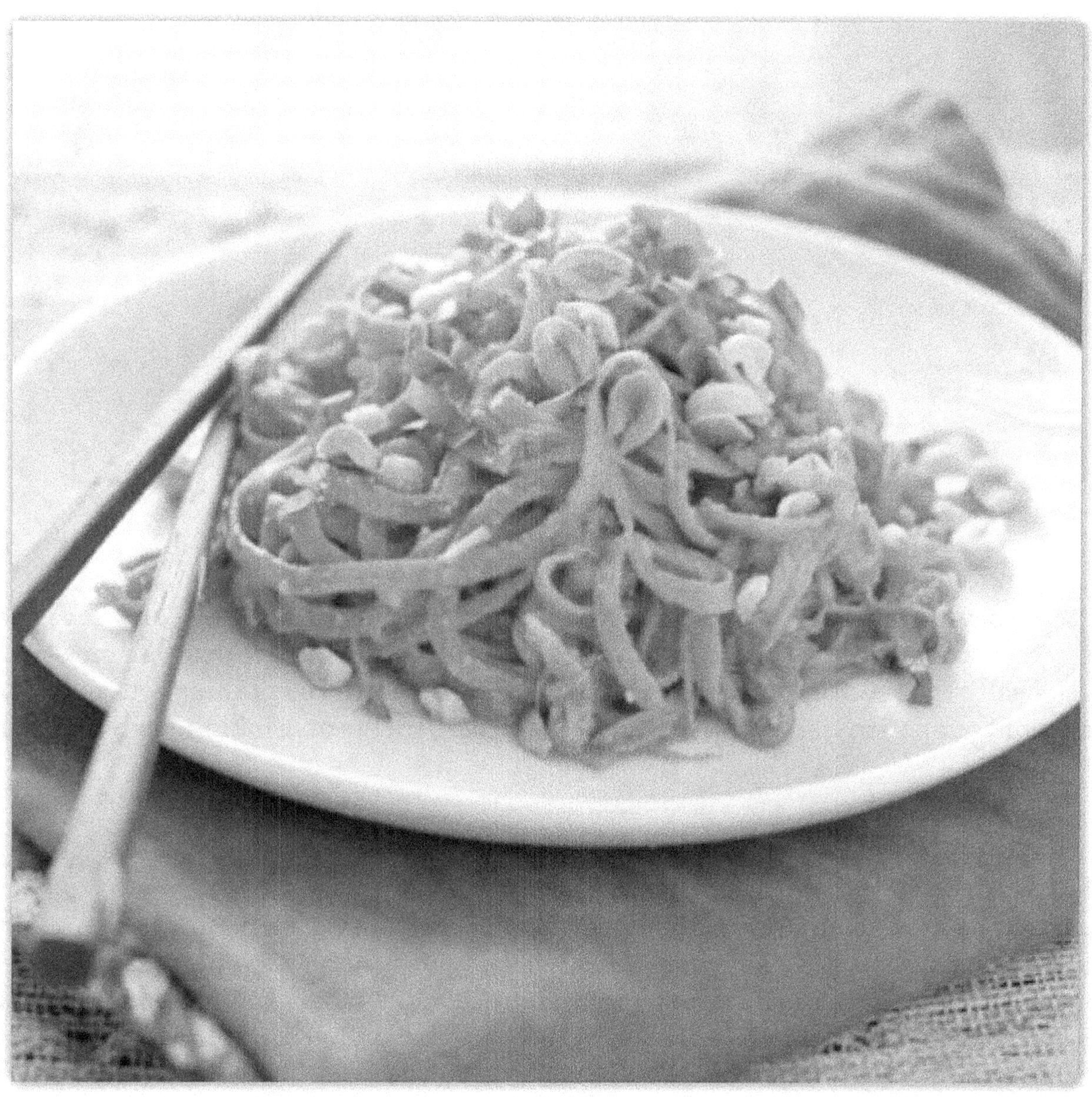

This is just one example of how you can make veggie noodles using zucchini, cucumber and carrots. This shows that you can enjoy raw veggie pastas as a filling snack.

The purpose of giving ideas for snacks is to motivate you. You will know that you don't have to eat vegetables in a not-so-fun way. Make your snack time interesting by trying out these ideas and creating your own dishes along the way. Share these healthy snack ideas as much as you can. You'll fall in love with this clean and lively way of eating!

◆ ◆ ◆

CHAPTER 6

What to do After the Cleanse?

You have done an amazing job in going through the full cleanse. Enjoy your success and rock the new outfits you once coveted. Now is the time to get your life on a steady health track. Go on an adventure with your friends and do something you couldn't do because of your health issues. You will surely reap the benefits of drinking green smoothies for 10 days.

Right After the Cleanse

As you have been on a completely different diet from what you were used to, don't go straight back to your previous eating habits. Eating whole foods is not a good idea after the green smoothie cleanse. For three days, eat very light meals like salads and sautéed vegetables. Keep drinking one or two glasses of smoothies for breakfast or lunch. Listen to your body and feed yourself what's best for you.

For two days after the detox, have a smoothie for breakfast. Eat salad for lunch and have sautéed vegetables for dinner. On the third day, have a glass of smoothie for breakfast. For lunch, you can have lean meat like chicken or fish with salad. Add sautéed vegetables to your plate alongside chicken. If you start with whole foods straight away, you will feel bloated and sick.

After three days, you can eat whole foods but keep them light and healthy to avoid gaining all the weight back. You will not crave unhealthy food at this point after the detox which is a good thing. Keep drinking a glass of smoothie for breakfast because it will help you to stay slim and fit. You can change the routine by replacing one meal with a green smoothie every day.

Maintaining Weight Loss

Many people complain about gaining all the weight back when they go off a calorie restricting diet. This happens because you can't keep on depriving yourself from so many food choices out there. You can't keep on counting the calories and measuring the portions all the time. You can't ignore your hunger and cravings if you are not satisfied with the meals you are eating. If the diet doesn't allow you to feel full for a longer period of time, it doesn't work in the future. The result is, you go back to the same food choices you wanted to leave behind. You gain weight again and make more mistakes. Let's leave all that in the past and look towards the present and future.

Weight loss is not about physical transformation. It's more of an emotional and mental journey. You know that you should not go back to whole foods right after the 10 day cleanse. Once you have done that, you might be worried about maintaining your weight or losing more weight in the future. If that is the case, continue to lose one or two pounds every week. This is a healthy goal and it's doable. Eat clean and healthy meals. Add more protein to your diet. Drink one smoothie in place of a meal, if you want to lose one pound every week and two glasses of smoothie as a replacement meal if you want to lose two pounds.

If you ask me to define "eating clean and healthy", your main goal should be to eat more vegetables and fruits, more water, salads, lean proteins like fish and chicken, healthy fats and good carbs. Your body can easily digest and effectively use natural and organic foods unlike those highly processed foods that are high in sugar, salt and fat.

Moreover, having protein with every meal will help you in weight loss. Our body doesn't react to proteins with insulin spikes as it does when we take processed carbs. Protein promotes that feeling of fullness and satisfaction. Naturally, we don't get hungry very often and don't crave the jar of cookies that is right in front of us. The key to maintaining weight loss even after the green smoothie cleanse is to eat whenever you are hungry. But if you think that it's going to disturb your routine, eat three main meals and two snacks. It will help you in losing weight quickly.

The full cleanse is meant for only ten days and no longer than two weeks. Your body needs a rest, otherwise you will be tired and you might harm your health. Eat a balanced diet that has a variety of healthy foods. It will boost your metabolism and you will feel energetic.

Besides having a good diet, PHYSICAL ACTIVITY is mentioned everywhere. Engaging in a physical activity doesn't mean that you have to spend hours in a gym. You can simply use stairs, walk more, and play your favorite game or sport. Add fun in physical activities if you have a busy schedule. You can take out a few minutes for simple yoga, rope jumping or having fun with a hula hoop. Discover your inner child who loves to play and have fun. If you enjoy what you are doing, it will help to manage stress and weight. Exercise and better sleep are two important aspects you should work on after the 10 day green smoothie cleanse to maintain a healthy weight and lifestyle. We talk about these common things but we need to incorporate them in our lives to achieve our health goals.

What to DO when you CAN'T Lose Weight?

Many people struggle with weight loss even if they are doing everything right. They eat a balanced diet, go through a detox and work out hard but the numbers on the scale are stuck or they keep on increasing. That is where you need to get your hormones checked. They play a huge role in your weight and overall health. Each hormone has a different role and how they work decides everything about our health.

Hormones that cause Weight Gain

These chemical messengers are very important in regulating different body functions including growth and development, hunger patterns, metabolism, mood and energy levels, sex drive and reproductive functions. Let's take a look at a few of them and see how you can bring balance in your body.

Leptin: It is a hormone that tells you to stop eating when you are full and it regulates your metabolism so that your body can burn fat whenever needed. Sleep plays a major role in keeping this hormone in balance. The Journal of Clinical Endocrinology and Metabolism states: "sleep duration plays an important role in the regulation of human leptin levels".

Eat at least two hours before going to sleep to keep this hormone in balance. You will not lose weight if this hormone doesn't tell you: "Stop eating honey! You've had enough".

The problem with hormonal imbalance is that if you have problem with one hormone, it can cause problems with other hormones too. It's like a domino effect. If your leptin levels aren't stable, it can affect other hormones like cortisol.

Cortisol: This hormone is synonymous with stress. Eating disorders are mostly related with tension and many people crave sugar and coffee when they are stressed out. When you are worried, this hormone triggers a "fight or flight" response. High levels of cortisol causes fat storage and muscle breakdown. This slows down metabolism. Adding fuel to the fire, many people resort to "stress eating" and you gain weight as a result.

The fast paced life of the modern world along with financial or emotional problems increase cortisol levels and we are stuck in the vicious cycle of making poor choices about our health. Personally, I have found that yoga and connecting more with my inner thoughts and spiritual side has helped me to reduce stress. Getting out for a walk in the morning has also helped me. If you feel that you need support, take your closest people in confidence. Talk to a therapist or a support group to manage stress. Otherwise it can cause imbalance in another hormone called ghrelin.

Ghrelin: It is the "hunger hormone". If you have high levels of ghrelin, it causes extreme hunger and cravings. The increased levels of leptin and cortisol are related to poor sleep and stress. That is also the case with ghrelin. The 10 day green smoothie cleanse is designed to balance these hormones that play a major role in hunger.

If the detox doesn't work or you can't lose any more weight after the detox, then you need to consider insulin resistance and the problems associated with it. One of the most common hormonal issues women are facing today is Poly Cystic Ovarian Syndrome, commonly known as PCOS. However, you need to visit a doctor to be sure about any hormonal problem. Let's take a look at insulin and what role it plays in our body.

Insulin: Insulin plays an important role in metabolizing glucose in the blood. It transports glucose to muscles and some of it is stored in the liver as glycogen. The extra glucose is stored as fat in our body. You see how important it is to maintain a healthy weight. If you eat sugar and processed carbs, you need more insulin to deal with all this food. This can sometimes affect ovaries in women and lead to weight gain and diabetes in men and women both.

Research shows that women with PCOS suffer with Beta cell dysfunction. These cells detect glucose in the blood and use it for energy. If you have PCOS, these cells produce more insulin than required. So, more glucose is stored up as fat instead of being used up for energy. This explains a lot of your problems including weight gain, increased levels of testosterone and difficulty in conceiving naturally.

However, there is a bright side. Besides conventional medication, doctors now agree that increased physical activity and managing insulin levels by eating carefully can resolve most of your problems. This 10 day green smoothie cleanse will give you a jump start and you can see improvements in your overall health but do consult a doctor before going through the green smoothie cleanse.

ESTROGEN:

Everything in our bodies is so interrelated that we can see a chain of reactions when there is disruption in any single element. Take a look at estrogen, a hormone that gives women their feminine features. At normal levels, it keeps you thin by helping insulin do its job. When estrogen levels increase than the normal limit, your beta cells are strained and you become insulin resistant. So, your body stores more insulin as fat and you gain weight as a result.

Taking less fiber and eating meat of animals that have been raised with an overload of antibiotics, steroids and toxins in their feed increase estrogen levels. To control your estrogen levels, eat more vegetables and increase your fiber intake. Out of all treatments and advice, this one is the simplest. Your aim should be to get 35-45 grams of fiber every day. If you are eating less fiber, add 5 grams more fiber every day to avoid digestive problem.

Messed up hormones make you feel weak, mentally disturbed, guilty, and you have low confidence and self-esteem. You feel that you are not in control of your body and mind. Consulting a physician is one way to go about this health issue that eats you up every day. Take control of your life by balancing one hormone at a time through lifestyle changes. The topic of women and weight loss is discussed over and over again but what many people fail to say is that it's not simply about weight loss. It's about feeling satisfied and happy with yourself, your health and your life. It's YOU who matter the most! When you feel strong and tranquil, you can focus on other important things in life: your hopes, dreams, aspirations and purpose.

Some Tips for Natural Weight loss and Fitness

Natural weight loss and fitness gets easy once you start taking small steps and make some changes in the way you eat. Here are a few useful tips for you:

- As I have been stressing on vegetables again and again, especially **BIG salads**, you will experience the amazing benefits of leafy greens and other colorful vegetables in your salad. You can use simple salad dressing like olive oil or lemons to make it tasty. Put a little fruit and red kidney beans in there to make it pop. Sometimes a boiled egg goes very well with the salad.

- **One smoothie per day** should be your goal after the 10 day cleanse. It will boost your health in so many ways. Feel free to add flax seed, coconut oil, almond milk and chia seeds.

- **Nutrient rich foods** are better than eating foods with little to no nutrients. Instead of a burger, try baked fish with sautéed vegetables. You can make wise choices even when you hang out with friends. Look for good food in different cuisines to add variety to your food choices.

- **Eat protein** with every meal and balance your carbs with sea food or any lean protein.

- Three most harmful elements in food are **salt, sugar and trans-fat**. In a BBC documentary, they tried to uncover the truth behind the addiction of processed foods. Their research revealed that a combination of salt, sugar and trans-fat makes these foods addictive and cause weight problems. Even at home, try to use less salt and trans-fat. Avoid sugar and use natural alternatives like fruits, especially dates, stevia, honey and maple syrup.

- **Eat red meat but not more than two times a week**. Instead, go for fish, sea food, poultry, vegetables, beans and nuts to get good fats.

- **Eating more fiber** helps with constipation, heart conditions, diabetes and many other diseases. You will naturally get fiber from vegetables, fruits, oats and whole grains. You can also use psyllium husk as a fiber supplement.

- **Eat snacks between meals**. To boost your metabolic function, eat three main meals and healthy snacks in between. After having a smoothie or a healthy breakfast, eat a light snack. Then have a snack after lunch. This will keep you satisfied throughout the day and you won't crave other unhealthy foods.

- **Stay Hydrated** as water plays an important part in flushing out toxins from your body. Just remember one thing: drink water one hour before a meal and not during and after a meal. Drink water after one hour of having a meal. It will improve your digestion.

- **Herbal tea** is better than coffee and normal tea. You can use any kind of herbal tea and I have also given a list of preferable herbal teas in Chapter 2. They don't have that caffeine kick but they help in burning fat more efficiently, improving hunger, lowering blood pressure and blood glucose levels, and improving digestion.

- **Let's not indulge in stress eating**. Whenever you are stressed or you want to hide your feelings by eating, stop yourself for a minute. Think about engaging yourself in a useful activity like cycling, painting, writing, spending time with a friend or reading a book. It's important to differentiate between physical hunger and hunger controlled by your feelings. Only then you can stop yourself from making mistakes about your health.

10 day green smoothie cleanse is not just about a change in your diet for 10 days. The real goal is to prepare yourself for making good changes in your life and the lives of your loved ones.

◆ ◆ ◆

CHAPTER 7

Making Smart Food Choices for Weight loss

Remember that the 10 day green smoothie cleanse is NOT a diet. It is simply a way to jump start weight loss and restore good health. If you want to try it again after a gap, you can but you can't expect the same dramatic weight loss. However, you can try the modified cleanse if you feel that you are not losing any more weight. This modified cleanse is also designed for those who are afraid that they can't stick with the full 10 day cleanse, can try this modified cleanse. The basic purpose of this cleanse is to get your body ready for the full cleanse. Even if that is not your goal, the modified cleanse helps you to detox. You will lose weight but the results will be a bit slower. Expect to lose 5 pounds or a bit more in 10 days.

Basic Guidelines for Modified Cleanse

1. DRINK TWO SMOOTHIES per day in place of your meals. Drink green smoothies for breakfast and lunch and eat a good healthy meal for dinner. You can have sautéed vegetables, salad, and a lean protein. Eating baked or grilled chicken or fish is a good idea. This way, you can get protein and improve your metabolism to lose weight.

2. Eat the same SNACKS allowed for the full cleanse. Take ideas from Chapter 5.

3. STAY HYDRATED and drink at least 8 glasses of water every day.

4. HERBAL TEA is so much helpful in the detox process. Drink any herbal tea of your choice before breakfast.

Just like the full cleanse, it's better to do it for only 10 to 14 days and not longer than that.

The long-term solution to weight loss as always is eating "clean" and I would like to add "make smart food choices". Let's see what these "smart" food choices are.

SMART Food Options and Not-so-Smart Choices

We all know some basics about what a healthy diet looks like. It is shown in a very general and textbook kind of way. The general guidelines usually start like this: a healthy plate consists of carbohydrates, proteins and vegetables. Fruits, dairy and nuts should be part of the diet. BUT what on earth should we eat if we need to lose weight and stay slim? If you try asking from your friends everyone will give you a different answer. Even if you do some research, you will get bombarded with so many different diets and all have a different set of rules. Some say fats are bad, cut out all of them. While some argue that we should eat more healthy fats. There are low-carb diets, protein diets, vegetarian, and some focus more on fruits. All these diets have a different approach towards food and nutrition. All of them have their own merits.

Tilting the weight on just one side of the scale is not the answer. BALANCE is the key to good health and harmony in your body and mind. Keeping that in mind, here is a list of foods you should eat to lose weight and foods you should avoid if you don't want to gain weight.

> **Vegetables**: *Eat all dark leafy greens, avocados, asparagus, broccoli, cauliflower, cabbage, cucumbers, celery, carrots, collard greens, kale, lettuce, ginger, green beans, onions, mushrooms, olives, parsley, mint, bell peppers, tomatoes, zucchini, peas, sweet potatoes, spinach*

Although all vegetables are good but there are vegetables that cause weight gain. These include white potatoes, corn, red potatoes and plantains.

> **Fruits:** *If you don't have a weight problem or you are not a diabetic, then you can eat all fruits. However, if you have any of these health issues, consume low-sugar fruits like blueberries, blackberries, cranberries, grapefruit, lemons, strawberries, apple and raspberries.*

Eating canned and dried fruits is not a smart food choice. Also, don't go for those tempting processed fruit snacks.

> **Meats**: *Eating mostly fish and sea food is a smart choice for weight loss. These include calamari, catfish, halibut, cod, crabmeat, clams, bass, sardines, shrimp, lobster, herring, chicken, turkey, trout, tuna, salmon etc. There might be other healthy*

lean meat options depending on where you live.

Meats you should avoid include bacon, sausage, beef jerky, hot dog, salami and fried meat.

> ***Dairy****: Almond milk, goat's milk, coconut milk, camel's milk, oat milk and eggs. Do note that camel's milk is one of those beneficial dairy products which helps in managing insulin, boosting immunity and helps in dealing with allergies like lactose intolerance.*

Avoid regular cow milk, cheese, cream cheese, cottage cheese, sour cream, powdered milk, and condensed milk.

> ***Grains (rice, pasta, bread)****: If you want to lose weight, it's best to watch the types of grains and carbs you are eating. Foods that support weight loss include brown rice, bulgur wheat, barley, quinoa, coconut flour, oats, barley and wild rice.*

You should avoid white flour, donuts, bagels, and all whites like pasta, bread and rice. Here white is not a friend; it's an enemy.

> ***Beans and Lentils****: Beans and lentils are mostly good as they are high in proteins. These include chickpeas, fava beans, all lentils, kidney beans, butter beans, peas, lima beans, black beans, pinto beans etc.*

You can eat all of them only if you boil them. However, canned beans with excess sodium, dried and refried beans are not an option if you want to lose the extra pounds.

> ***Nuts and Seeds****: Use unsalted nuts such as almonds, cashews, hazelnuts, pistachios, peanuts, walnuts etc. Seeds include flax seeds, chia seeds, pumpkin seeds, sunflower seeds, and sesame seeds.*

Avoid all sugar coated and salted nuts and seeds to reduce weight.

> ***Oils****: All fats and oils are not bad for health. Some are really good, such as olive oil, coconut oil, avocado oil, fish oil, sesame oil and flax seed oil.*

Vegetable oil, hydrogenated oil (trans-fat), bacon fat, margarine, and chicken fat cause weight gain, increase cholesterol levels, raise blood pressure and lead to stroke and heart diseases. Eating fried foods is also not a very smart choice, even if you choose healthy fats and oils for that. Use healthy fats and oils in moderate or small quantities while baking, grilling or sautéing vegetables and meats.

Sweeteners: You don't have to cut out all sweeteners to lose weight. Go for natural substitutes like stevia, agave nectar, and raw honey.

Try to avoid artificial sweeteners such as aspartame, acesulfame, saccharine, sucralose and neotame. These sweeteners are regulated by FDA but a study conducted on zero calorie drinks show that they cause more harm than good because they are processed and fake. They play with our taste buds and we crave more sweets. There are other factors involved and it was found that the consumption of these sweeteners contributed to long-term weight gain and even cancer.

Avoid these sweeteners at all costs if you want to stay healthy and slim: white sugar, brown sugar, corn syrup, raw sugar and fruit juice concentrate.

Spices and Seasonings: Most of the spices don't contribute to weight gain and they make food taste good. Use black pepper, chili peppers, cilantro, turmeric, ginger, garlic, apple cider vinegar, cinnamon, nutmeg, saffron, cardamom, onion, rosemary etc.

Use spices and seasonings from different cuisines but don't go for recipes that require mayonnaise, Worcestershire sauce, ketchup and MSG. Stop even buying these things if you are serious about weight loss, even if a family member loves these condiments.

Snacks: You have read a lot about snacks in this book and even seen a few recipes and examples. Snacking on healthy foods like fresh vegetables and fruits, lightly salted popcorn, unsweetened peanut and almond butter, hard boiled eggs, organic and unsweetened dark chocolate, plain yoghurt (plain Greek yoghurt is preferable), and nuts and seeds are the best not only during the green smoothie cleanse but also as a part of your everyday diet.

STAY AWAY from sugary treats we can't resist: donuts, cakes, candies, and ice cream. Fried foods that are very tempting include French fries, fried wings, and many other snacks are not important than your health.

Drinks: Nothing beats the importance of distilled or spring water. But if you get

> *bored with simple water and smoothies try adding slices of fruits and vegetables like oranges, apricots, strawberries, mint, lemons, watermelon or cucumber to plain purified water. There is something that will be more fun. Put crushed fruit pulp in an ice cube tray, any fruit you like. Then add water and freeze. You will really enjoy the flavor from these colorful ice cubes*

Other smart options include fresh fruit juice without added sugar, coconut water, and herbal teas.

For soda lovers who want to go through the detox and stay healthy, can make a fake one at home. It's not the real thing but it'll taste better than the usual soda you drink. Add a few slices of lemon and lime and add them in sparkling water with a little stevia-based sweetener. Remember to use a very "little" amount of sweetener. However, it's better if you add flavor to plain purified water to avoid gas and bloating.

Unhealthy drinks include sodas, store bought juice, sports drinks, beer and other alcoholic drinks.

> ***Cooking Methods:*** *Go for baking, boiling, poaching, sautéing, stir frying, grilling, steaming and pressure cooking.*

Never choose to fry, barbecue, and char your food. It will lose all nutritional value and you will not be able to achieve your weight loss goal.

Add Superfoods in Smoothies

Adding superfoods in smoothies increase the amounts of minerals, vitamins, fiber and other nutrients to help you manage any health condition, boost your energy levels and keep you fit and active. They have long-term benefits and also help in losing weight after the 10 day green smoothie cleanse. Make them part of your lifestyle and you will feel the powerful impacts of these superfoods in your life.

- ➤ Aloe Vera: Known for its anti-fungal and anti-bacterial properties. Also good for skin
- ➤ Avocado: a good source of healthy fats
- ➤ Chia seeds: Promote weight loss and manage hunger
- ➤ Raw chocolate: It has anti-aging properties.
- ➤ Coconut oil: Good for burning fat. Also a natural beauty treatment.
- ➤ Flax seed: For boosting immunity
- ➤ Ginger: aids in digestion

➤ Pomegranate: Promotes heart health

➤ Turmeric: Healing properties

➤ Yoghurt: A probiotic that is important for gut health

Making smart choices and being patient about any visible changes in your physique is the right approach towards your health goals. It takes time to drop pounds and lose dress sizes. Commit to improve your health first and stop fidgeting about the numbers. Don't jump in the challenge for 10 days only. Be prepared for making life-long changes in your thinking and everything about your health and the happiness of people around you. If you want to lose 20 pounds, set your goal for 2 or 3 months. Doing things naturally takes time and it requires both patience and commitment. You can do it!

◆ ◆ ◆

CHAPTER 8

50 Sensational Green Smoothie Recipes

Smoothies are the real deal when it comes to having a diet that not only tastes delightful but also has great nutritional value. Made from green vegetables, fruits, natural herbs and all kinds of amazing elements, smoothies are a "must include" item in your diet.

The best thing about these recipes is that they only require some 'magical mixing' of ingredients and a little blending in your blender and voila! Knowing the benefits of green smoothies gives you an edge. You can include them in your everyday life and reap the benefits they have to offer. By adding variety and experimenting with your smoothies, you can adjust the taste and heartily enjoy them.

If you want to lose weight, there are weight loss recipes to help you with that. If you are committed to detox, there are a number of detox smoothies. Finally, one important thing we can't miss is how to stay active and boost our energy. So, dive in and try these sensational green smoothies!

The recipes in this book have been gathered from culinary experts and nutritionists who just love to experiment and create sensational smoothies. Also, these smoothies are very easy to make!

Weight Loss Smoothies

Achieving that perfect figure seems really hard. More importantly, reducing that undesired body fat seems even harder. The 10 day green smoothie cleanse will jump start weight loss. Then comes the question of losing more weight. The answer is not that complicated. Drink smoothies to lose weight! Here is a variety of smoothies which are easy to make and it's the best way to incorporate fresh fruits and vegetables in your diet. These smoothie recipes also provide you with the much needed monounsaturated fatty acids which aim to reduce belly fat. They are creamy, rich and perfect for breakfast, lunch or as a snack.

Super Veggie Smoothie:

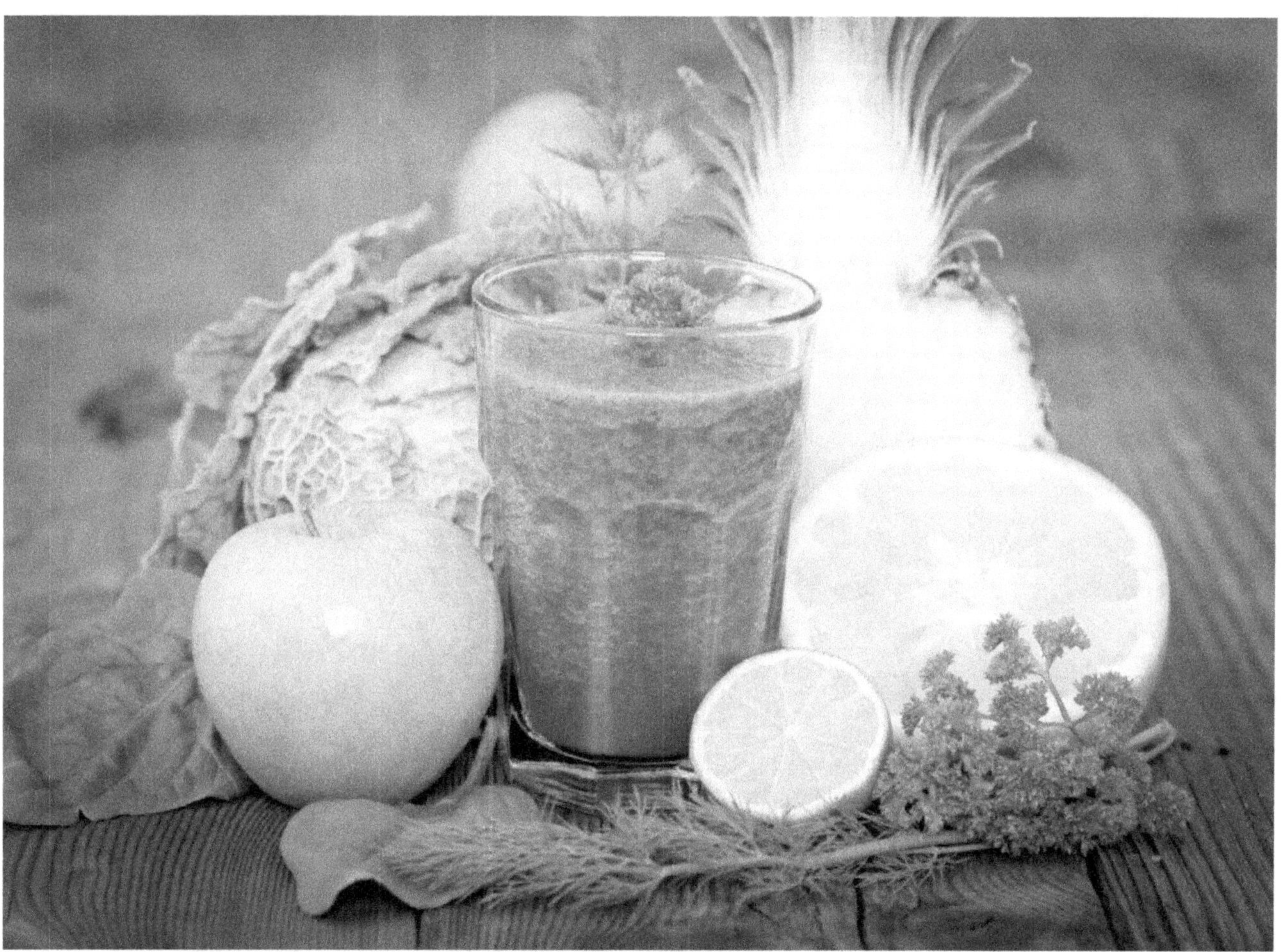

As broccoli is a very healthy vegetable, it is known as the 'Super Veggie.' With potassium, fiber, iron, vitamin C and vitamin K, it's quite high in nutrients. Paired with strawberry, it will rapidly reduce your weight by increasing your metabolism. This happens because it has more protein as compared to other vegetables.

Ingredients:
1) Broccoli florets - 1 cup
2) Strawberries – 1/2 cup
3) Chopped pineapple – 1/4 cup
4) Almond milk - 1 cup
5) Honey - 1 tsp

Blend everything and enjoy this nutritious smoothie. You don't like broccoli? Doesn't matter as the strawberries and pineapple will mask its taste and make the smoothie delicious.

Spinach with Berries Smoothie:

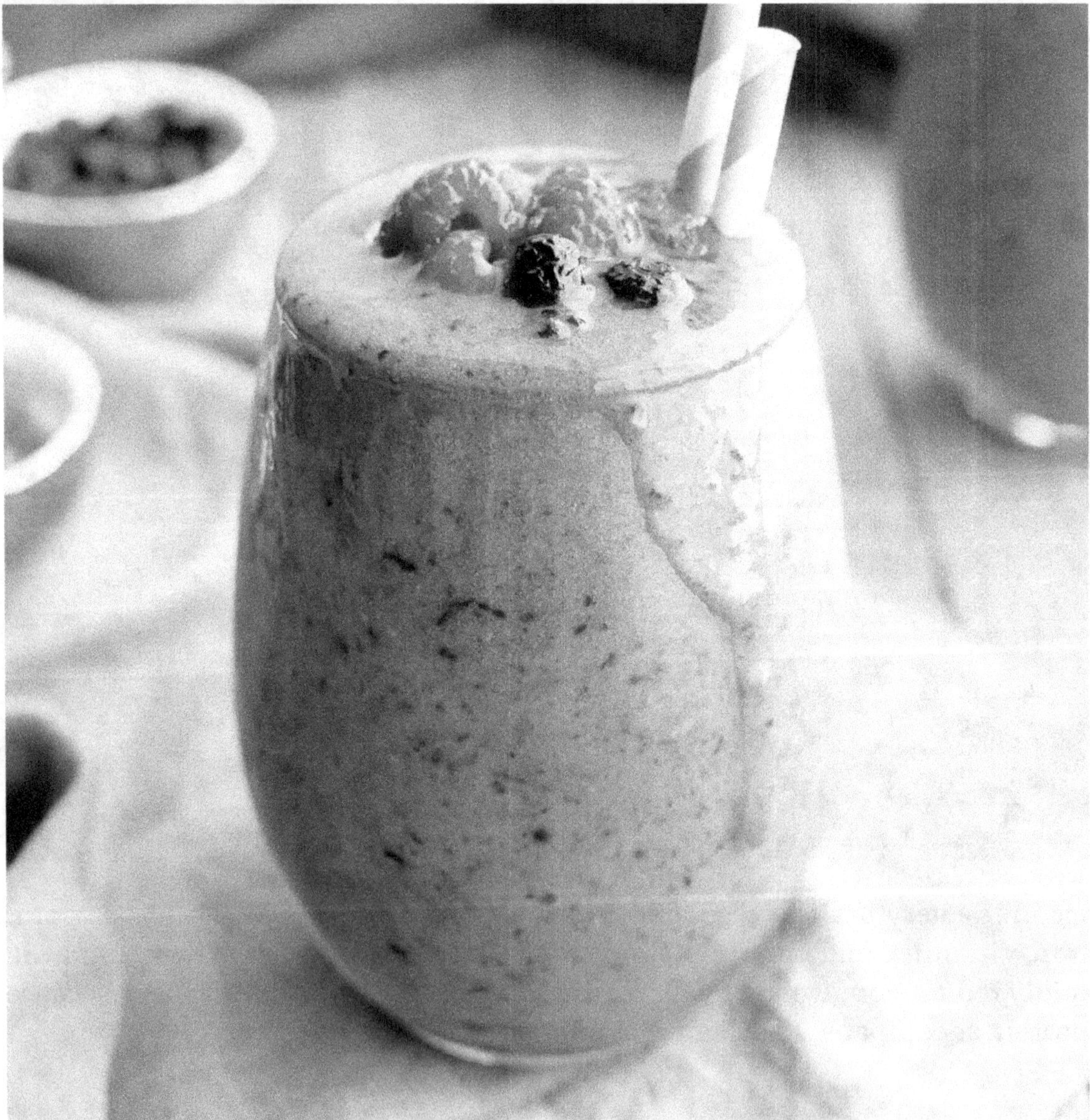

Spinach itself is enough to help you lose weight but when coupled with strawberries and berries, it will work miracles for you. This smoothie is packed with lots of vitamins and minerals our body needs.

Ingredients:
1) Spinach (fresh is preferable) – 1/4 cup
2) Frozen berries (blueberries and raspberries) - 2 cups
3) 5 sliced strawberries
4) Orange Juice – 1/2 cup
5) Plain yogurt - 1 cup

Blend the berries, strawberries, spinach, orange juice and yogurt until the mixture is smooth. You will get a creamy, purplish-pink colored drink full of berries that will aid in burning your fat.

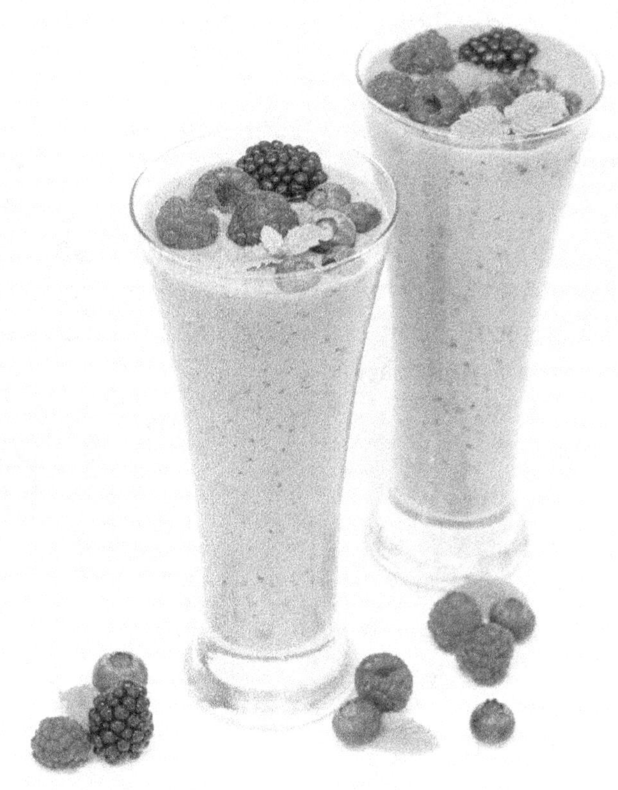

Peas Burst Smoothie:

With this smoothie, you will get a blast of health boosting nutrients. It contains nutrients that will fight your ever increasing weight. Sweet peas have more fiber and protein but only about 0.5g of fat. It's one of the healthiest foods in the world. One of the reasons of weight gain is continually eating without stopping. Chia seeds have soluble fibers that absorb water and expand the stomach. This will make you feel full so you won't eat more than required.

Ingredients:

1) Sweet peas - 1 cup
2) Blueberries – 1/2 cup
3) One banana
4) Almond milk - 1 cup
5) Chia seeds - 1 tbsp.
6) Honey – 1/2 tsp

Give everything a good whirl in a blender and savor this antioxidant drink for as long as you like.

Cocoa Cherry Smoothie:

The smoothie may not be green but it has spinach in it. Spinach makes this drink a potential source of iron, protein and various vitamins. Protein controls your appetite, which is really important when dieting. Did you know that cocoa and cherries have antioxidants to fight inflammation? How amazing is that!

Ingredients:

1) A handful of spinach
2) Unsweetened frozen cherries – 1/2 cup
3) Cocoa powder - 2 tsp
4) Frozen banana chunks – 1/4 cup
5) Chia seed - 2 tsp
6) Almond extract – 1/4 tsp

Grind and mix well and you will get tasty chocolate cherry smoothie. If you like chocolate, you will love this one.

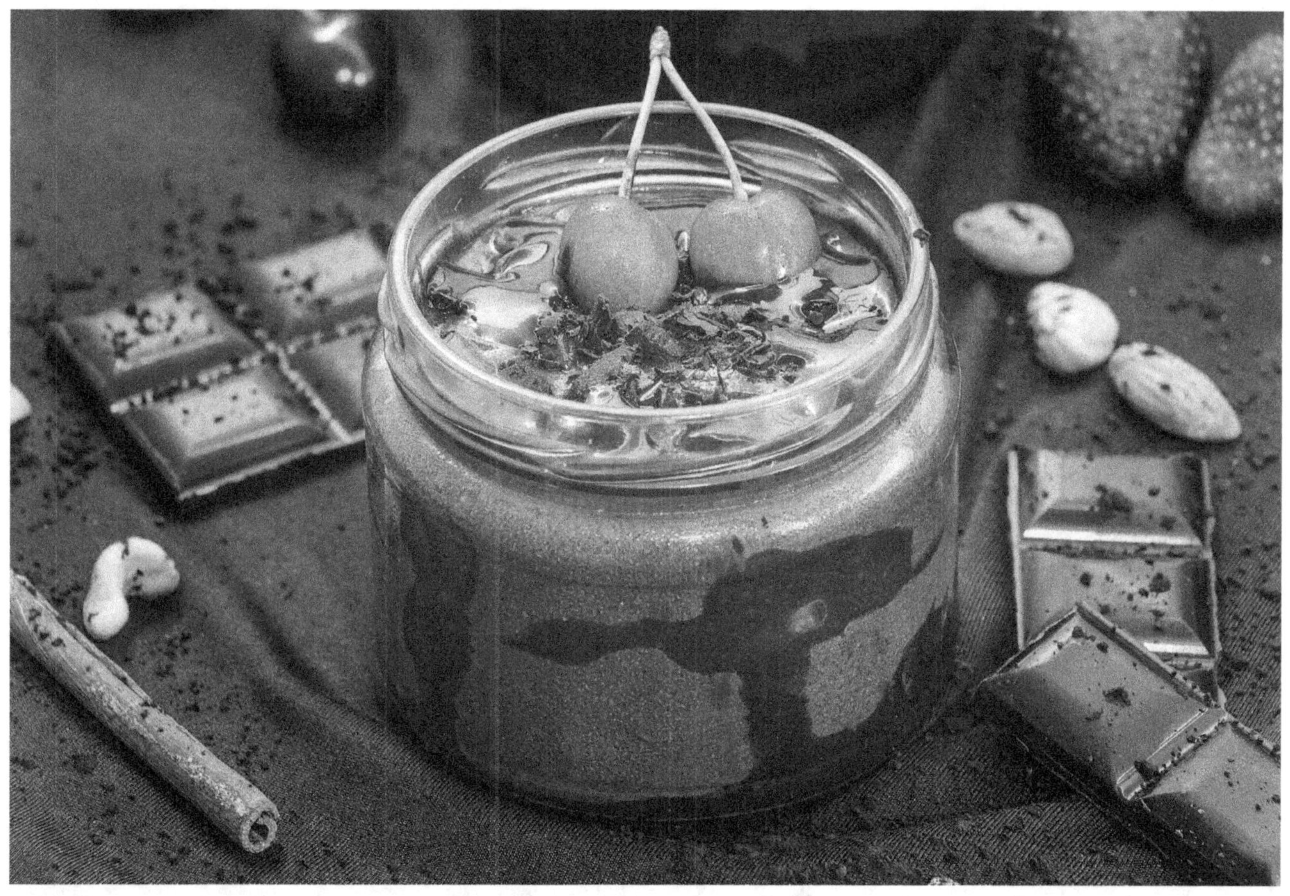

Kiwi with Lime Smoothie:

Kiwi and lime are the perfect couple. Kiwi is, after all, the champion of fruits when it comes to weight loss. It is low in calories and high in nutrients like calcium, iron, magnesium and potassium. Lime will burn your calories and aid the body in storing less fat.

Ingredients:
1) Kiwi (peeled and chopped)
2) Lime Juice from half a lime
3) 1 pear
4) Purified Water - ¼ cup
5) Honey (optional) - 1 tbsp.
6) Ice cubes - 1 cup

Make a refreshing and cool smoothie/cocktail that is fit for summer.

Raspberry Avocado Smoothie:

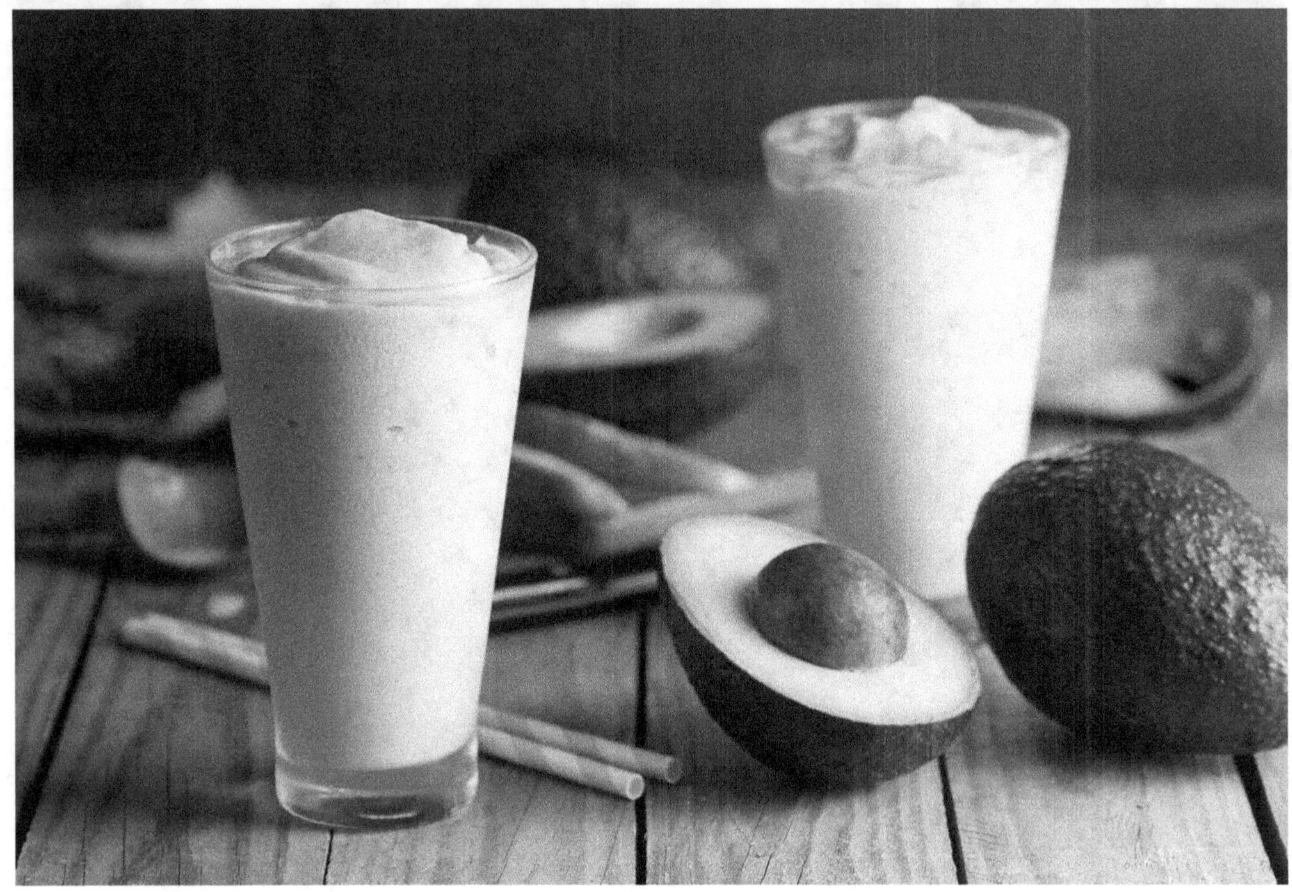

With spinach, raspberries, avocado and chia seeds, this smoothie packs a punch. It will compel the body to oxidize more fat because of iron and counter cortisol, the

stress hormone which increases belly fat reserves.

Ingredients:

1) Frozen raspberries - 1 cup

2) 2 handfuls of spinach
3) Half avocado
4) Chia seeds - 1 tbsp.
5) Half banana
6) Unsweetened almond milk – 3/4 cup

Blend them smoothly and relish this epic weight loss smoothie.

Kale and Berry Smoothie:

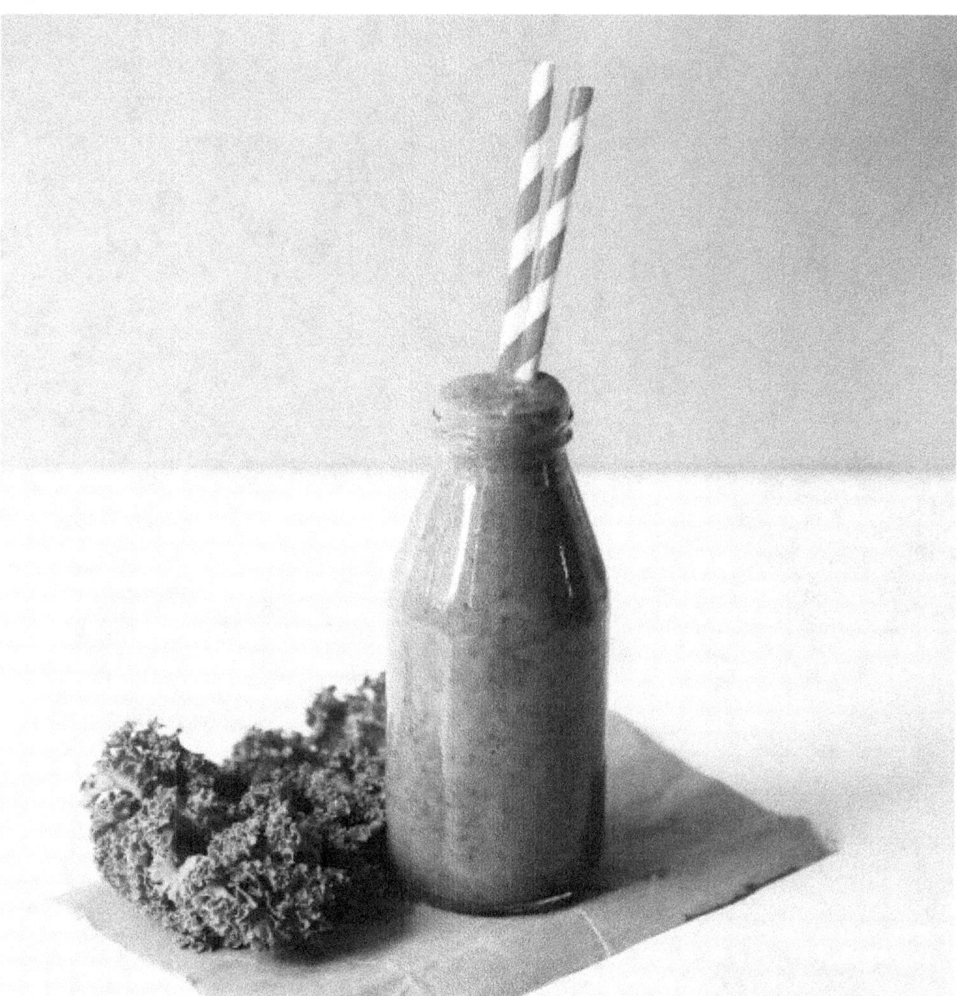

This kid friendly and flavorful smoothie has vitamin C and antioxidants which come from cherries and berries. It's also low in calories. Say a bold NO to weight gain with it!

Ingredients:

1) Fresh kale - 1 cup
2) Cherries – 1/2 cup
3) Blueberries – 1/2 cup
4) Almond milk - 1 cup
5) Honey - 2 tsp

Give all the ingredients a nice spin and enjoy this kale smoothie flavored with cherries and berries.

TIP: Use fresh fruit, the smoothie will be more nutritious and delicious.

Honeydew Melon Green Smoothie:

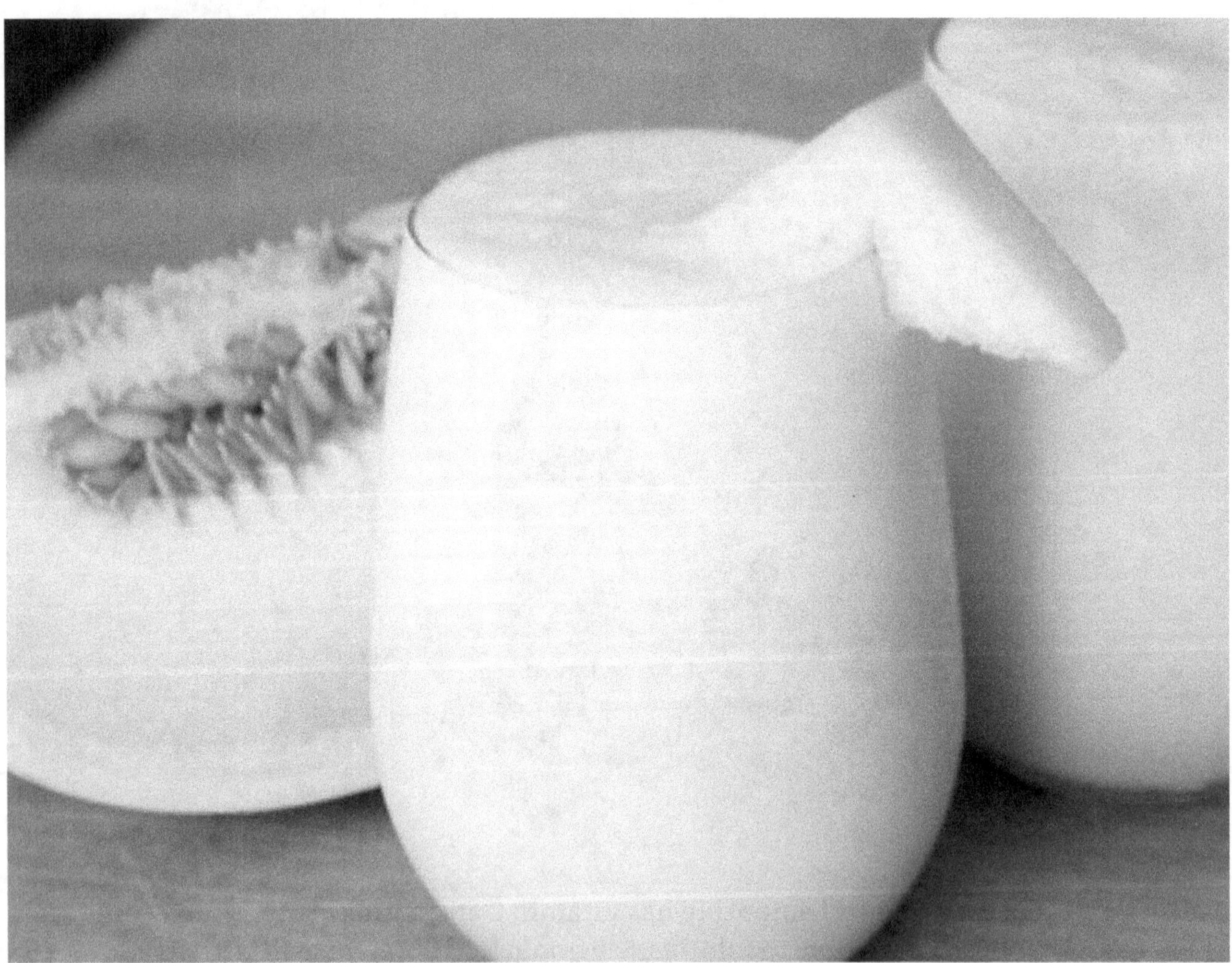

It is a combination of green vegetables like mint, cucumber and dandelion greens. Dandelion greens have stolen the spotlight from the other greens as it is rich in dietary fiber, protein and minerals such as iron and calcium. This smoothie will freshen you up as it has both cucumber (watery) and mint (coolness). You will be surprised but cucumber is known to boost silica, manganese, folate and magnesium levels in the body. All of these are essential trace elements needed to prevent deficiencies.

Ingredients:

1) Honeydew melon cut into cubes - 2 cups
2) Half peeled cucumber
3) 1 frozen banana
4) Dandelion greens - 3 cups
5) 6 mint leaves
6) Lime juice - 1 tsp
7) Unsweetened almond milk - 1 cup

Blend the liquid ingredients first and then add the greens and the banana. Pour the tantalizing and health boosting drink and enjoy!

Watermelon Red Smoothie:

Not only will this smoothie reduce your weight, it will

also keep you hydrated. One of the perks of water is that

it suppresses appetite, something that is really important if you want to lose weight.

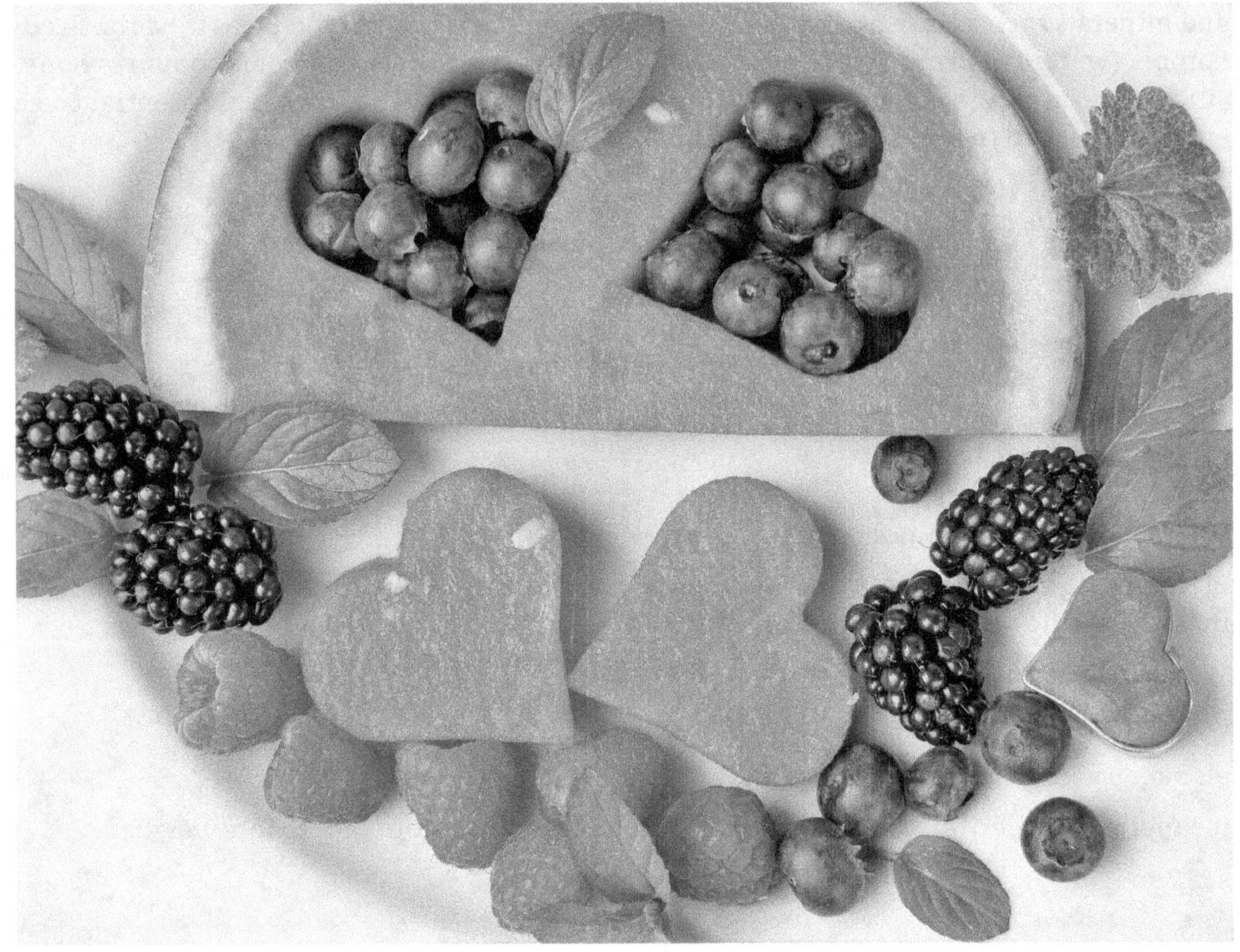

Ingredients:

1) Watermelon cubes - 2 cups
2) Lime juice - 1 tbsp.
3) Frozen strawberries - 1 cup
4) 6 ice cubes
5) Honey (optional) - 2 tsp

Blend this superb smoothie but make sure to use seedless watermelon or you will end up biting seeds in every sip you take.

Four Greens Smoothie

Just as the name suggests, this smoothie is made with four green vegetables. These veggies will help in controlling blood sugar level, prevent constipation, and restrain your appetite which is very important for weight loss. It also keeps you hydrated. More water will aid in reducing your water weight (mass of the water in a person's body) as more water will be excreted from the body.

Ingredients:

1) A handful of kale
2) A handful of spinach
3) Cucumbers (sliced) – 1/4 cup
4) Raw parsley – 1/4 cup
5) Frozen strawberries – 5
6) Half lemon
7) Almond milk - 1 cup

Grind everything in a blender until no chunks are left. Try this smoothie for losing weight.

Green Ginger and Date Smoothie

Cucumber is the star of healthy vegetables. It's filled with benefits as it decreases the risk of cancer and im

proves the digestive, mental and cardiac health. Plus, it gives you good breath.

Ingredients:

1. Peeled cucumber – 1/2 cup
2. One quarter of an avocado (peeled)
3. Crushed ginger – 1/2 tsp
4. Baby spinach - 1 cup
5. Two dates
6. Lemon juice from 1 lemon
7. Hemp seeds - 2 tbsp.
8. Water - 1 ½ cups
9. Sea salt - to taste
10. Parsley for garnishing (optional)

Remove the stones of avocado and dates. You can even use ice cubes if you like cold smoothie. Blend all the ingredients together and drink this healthy, weight loss green smoothie.

Coconut Mint Lime Smoothie:

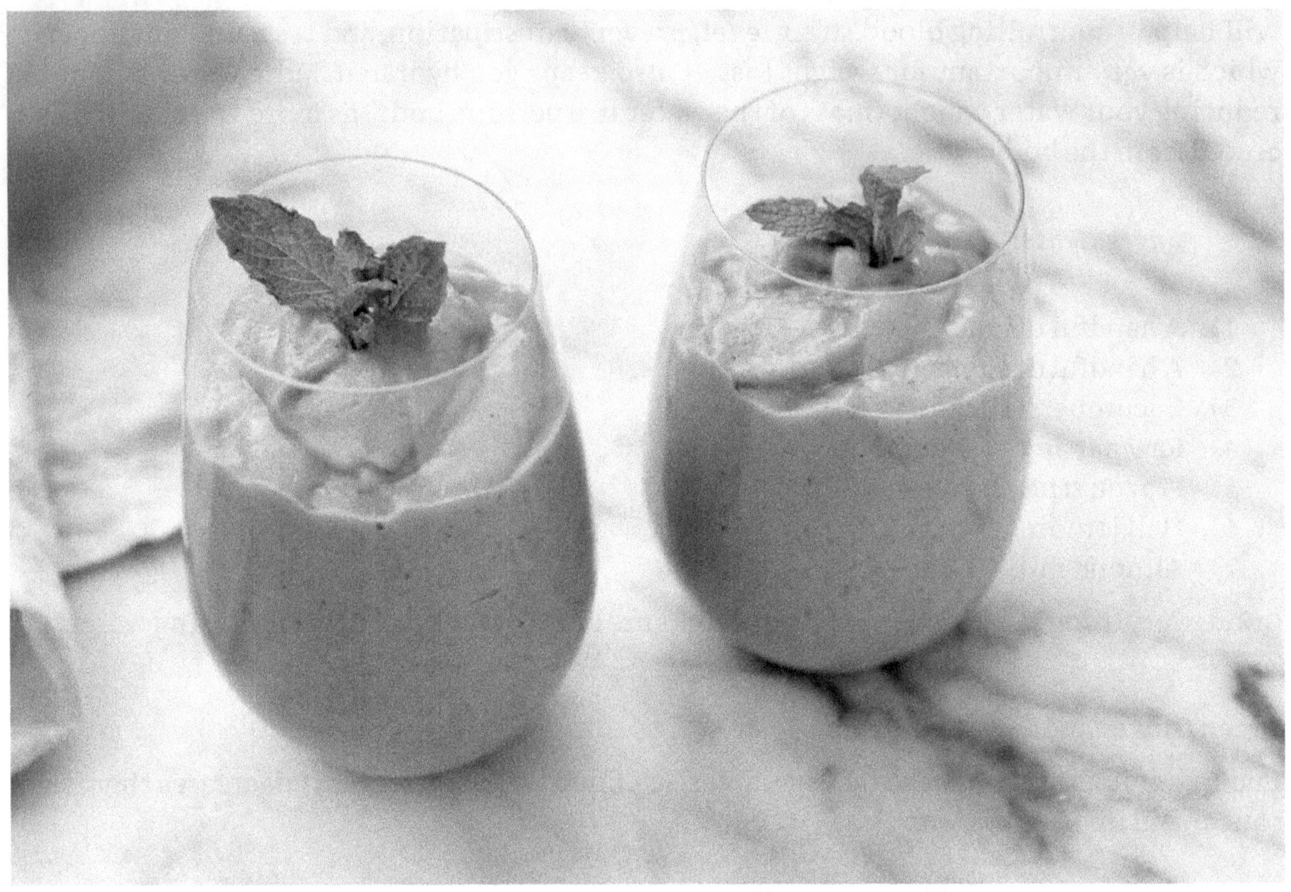

Mint can help you lose a pound or two as it aids in digestion. When digestion is efficient, then all nutrients are readily absorbed and waste is more easily removed. In this, no extra stuff remains to become part of the body. Also, coconut water (easy on the stomach) and lime juice are quite helpful as they burn excess fats.

Ingredients:

1) Raw spinach – 1/2 cup
2) Coconut water – 3/4 cup
3) Lime juice from two fresh limes
4) A handful of fresh mint
5) 1 sliced banana

First, blend the coconut water, mint and spinach. Then, add the lime juice and banana and blend until the smoothie is nice and smooth. Top it with tart lime and enjoy!

Spinach with Grapefruit Smoothie:

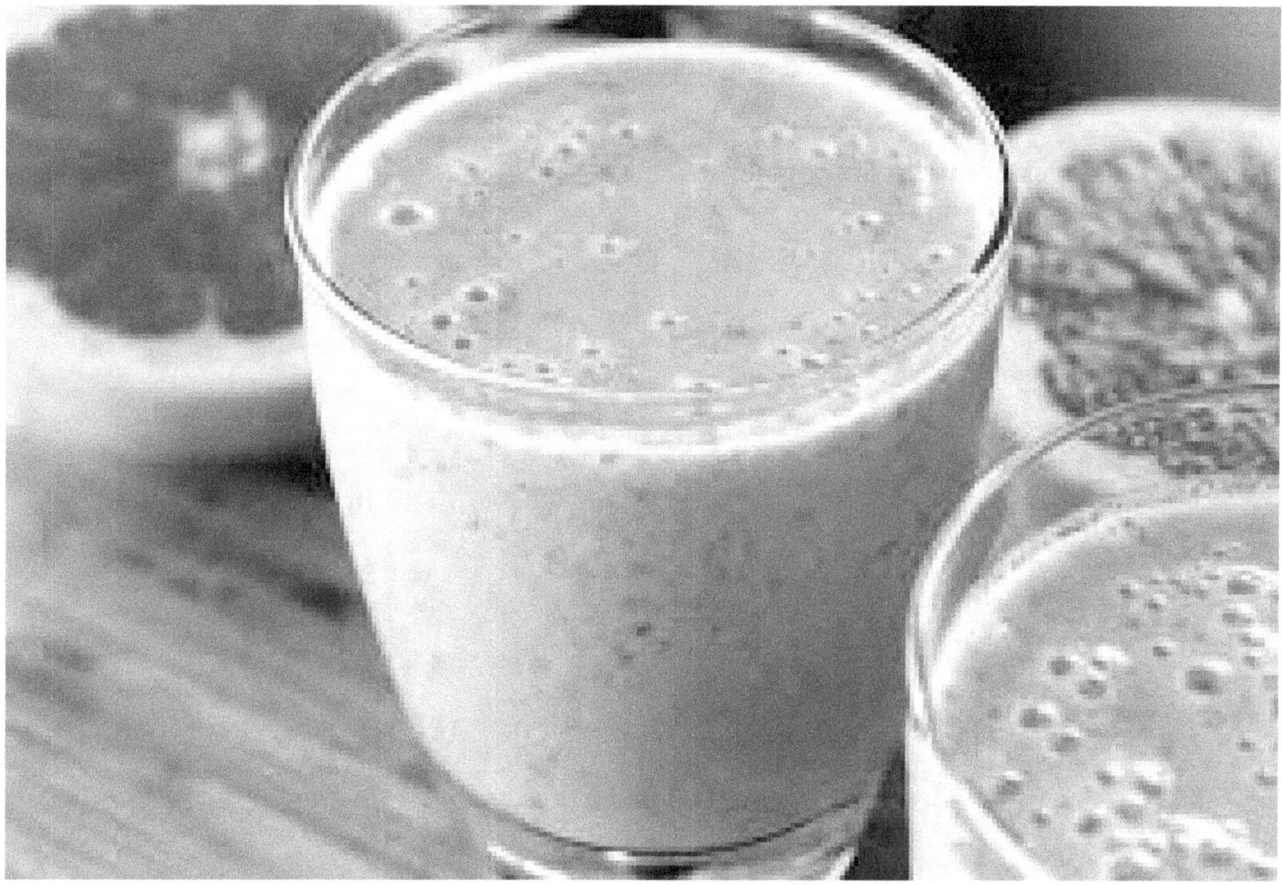

With Spinach, apple and banana this smoothie is abundant in nutritional value. Spinach reduces the desire for food and burns fat at a fast rate. On the other hand, grapefruit has a lot of minerals and vitamins that the body needs. These nutrients will lead to a healthy heart and immune system and even reduce weight to some extent.

Ingredients:
1) Spinach - 2 cups
2) 1 sliced banana
3) 1 grapefruit
4) 1 apple
5) Unsweetened almond milk or water – 1/2 cup

6) Ginger – 1/2 tsp
7) 2 ice cubes

Peel the apple, ginger and grapefruit. Then, separate the seeds of grapefruit and the core of apple. Blend everything together until the mixture is smooth and creamy. You can even use more banana or apple to make it sweeter and thick. It's completely up to you.

Strawberry Ginger Kiwifruit Smoothie:

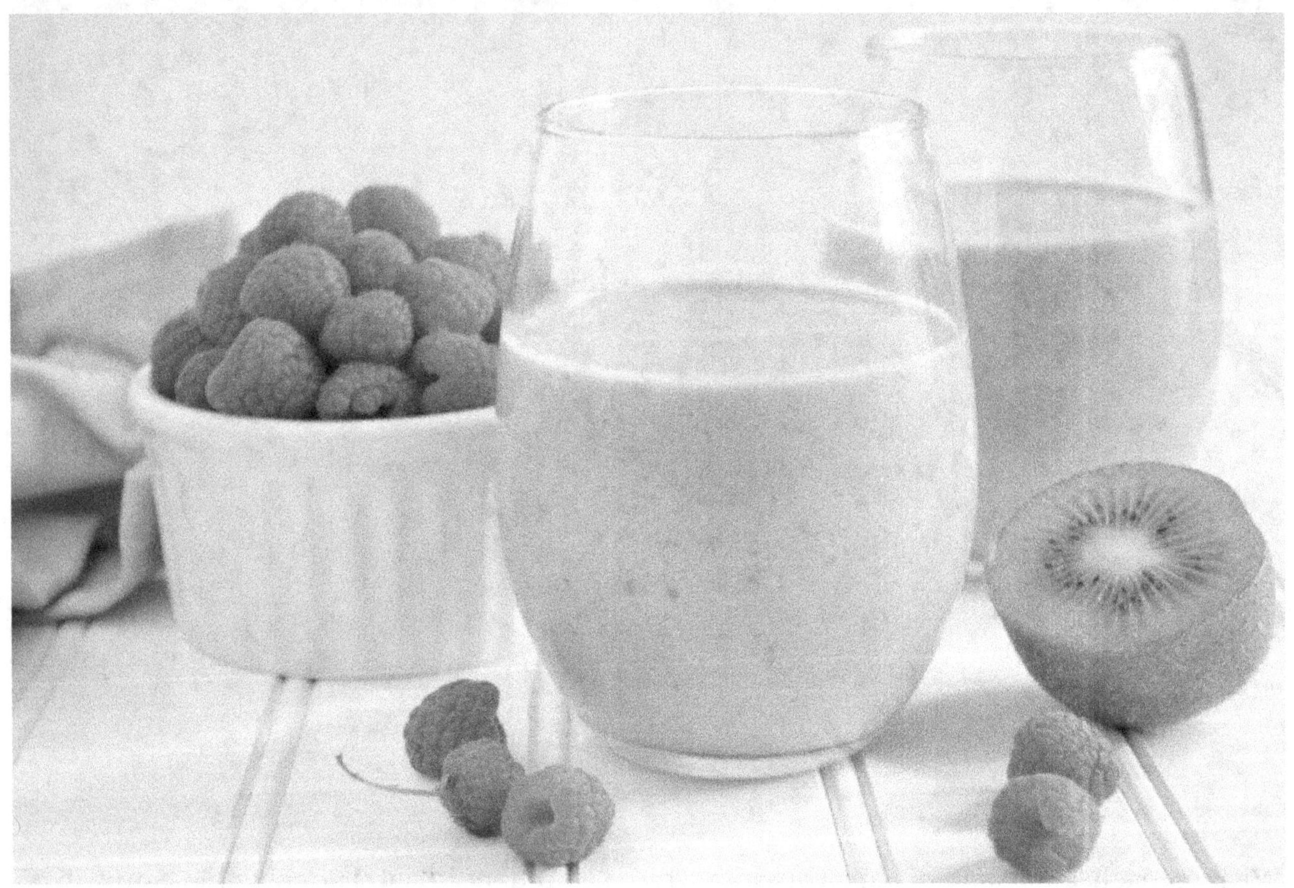

Strawberry and ginger are an excellent pair. Ginger will make you feel full while strawberry will control your sugar cravings. Anyone who wants to drop a few pounds should try this weight loss smoothie.

Ingredients:
1) Spinach – 1 cup

2) Crushed ginger - 1 tsp
3) Strawberries - 1 cup
4) 2 kiwis
5) Chia seeds - 1 tbsp.
6) Almond milk – 3/4 cup
7) 4 ice cubes

Blend spinach and ginger first. Slice strawberries and kiwis. Then add the rest of the ingredients in the blender, blend and sip this sweet smoothie.

Green Banana Smoothie:

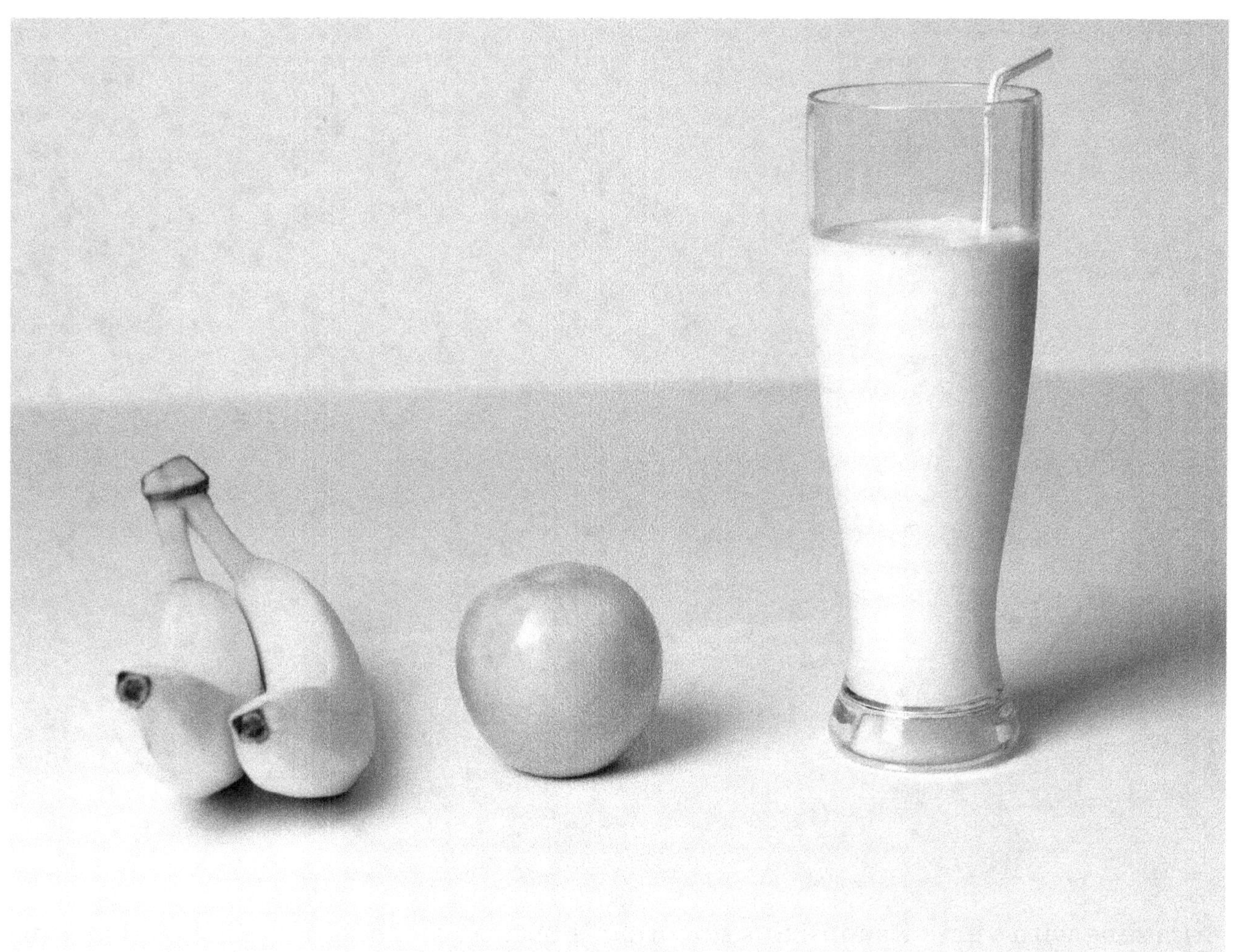

Banana is the powerhouse of fruits as it has got a lot of fiber to spare and is low in calories. Such fruits are known to lower weight. Coupled with kale - the green part - this smoothie will burn some belly fat and make \you healthy at the same time.

Ingredients:
1) Chopped kale leaves - 2 cups
2) One diced banana
3) Almond milk – 1/2 cup

Blend and enjoy this creamy and green smoothie. You can also add honey and ice cubes if you want. But remember to remove the stems and ribs of the kale leaves to get a fine creamy texture.

Fruity Kiwis Smoothie:

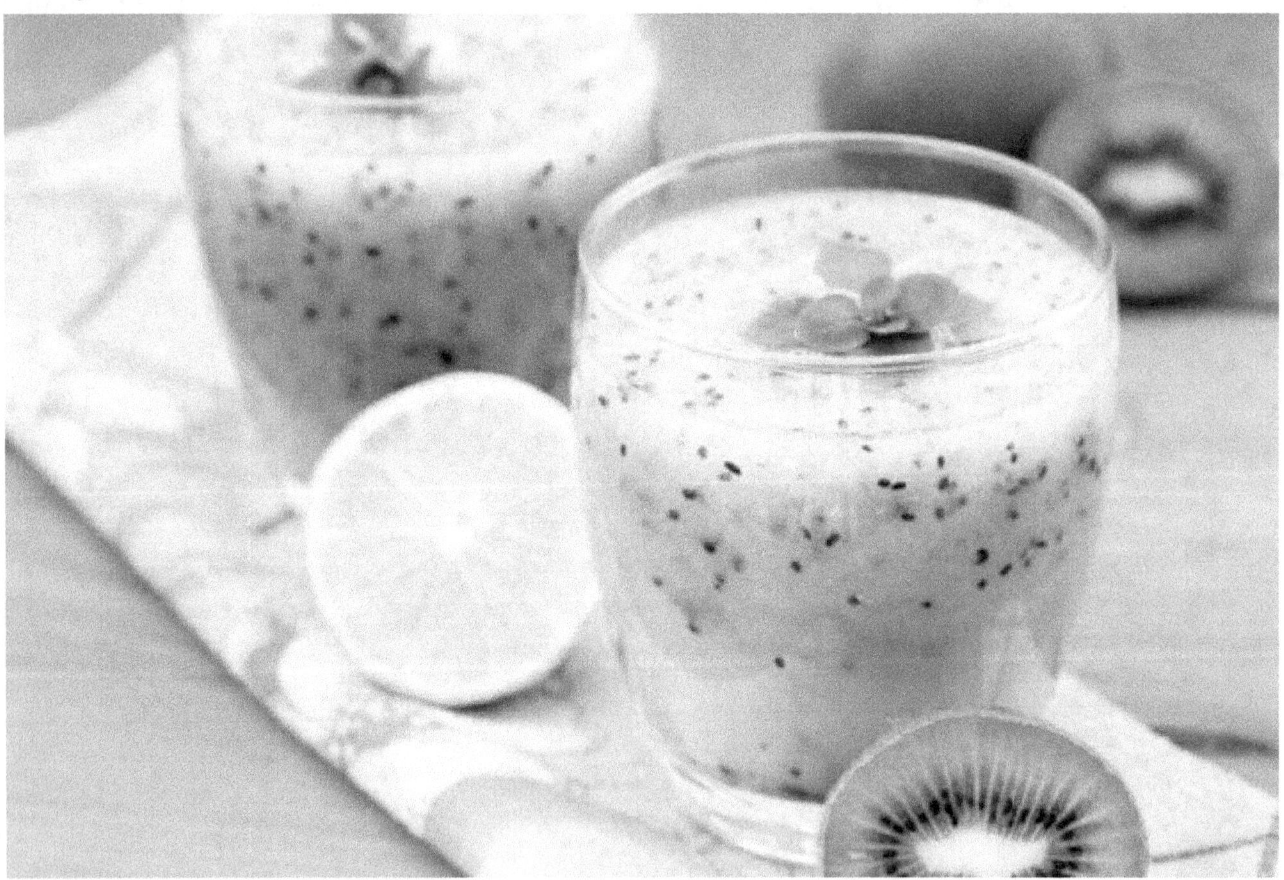

Brimming with vital vitamins, this smoothie is nutritious. These fruits help in lowering cholesterol and reduce belly fat.

Ingredients:

1) Spinach – 1 cup
2) Strawberries - 1 cup
3) Peaches (without the stone/pit) - 1 cup
4) 3 fresh kiwis (peeled and chopped)
5) Blueberries - ½ cup
6) Frozen bananas - 1 cup
7) Orange juice - ½ cup
8) Greek yogurt - 1 cup

Blend until the consistency of the mixture is smooth. You have to follow the recipe completely to get a fruity flavor.

Low Carb Smoothie:

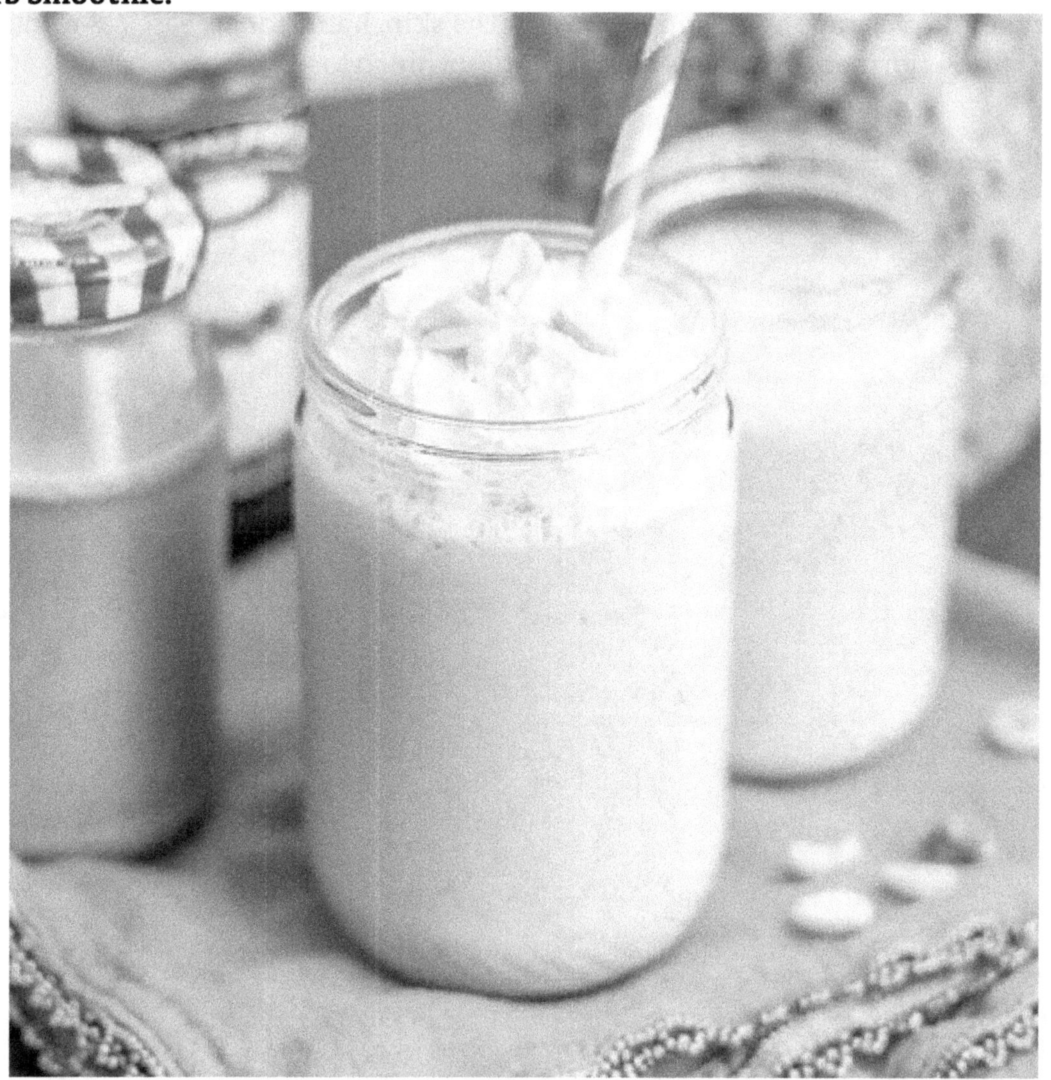

To reduce belly fat, it's better to eat vegetables and fruits with lower calories. Lettuce with dark green leaves and apple are the perfect for reducing weight. Lettuce is high in vitamins A and C which are important for the immune system. It has loads of water reserves and no cholesterol or fats in it. While the fiber in apples will boost your metabolism. Both of them will keep you full and content for a longer time so that you won't feel the need to munch on more food. Hence, your body will slim down.

Ingredients:
1) Lettuce - 1 bunch
2) Apple - 1
3) Honey – 1/2 tsp

Chop lettuce and grate apple without removing the skin. Blend for at least 7-8 minutes until a smooth paste is formed. Drink this fiber rich smoothie to lose weight.

Fuji Apple Smoothie:

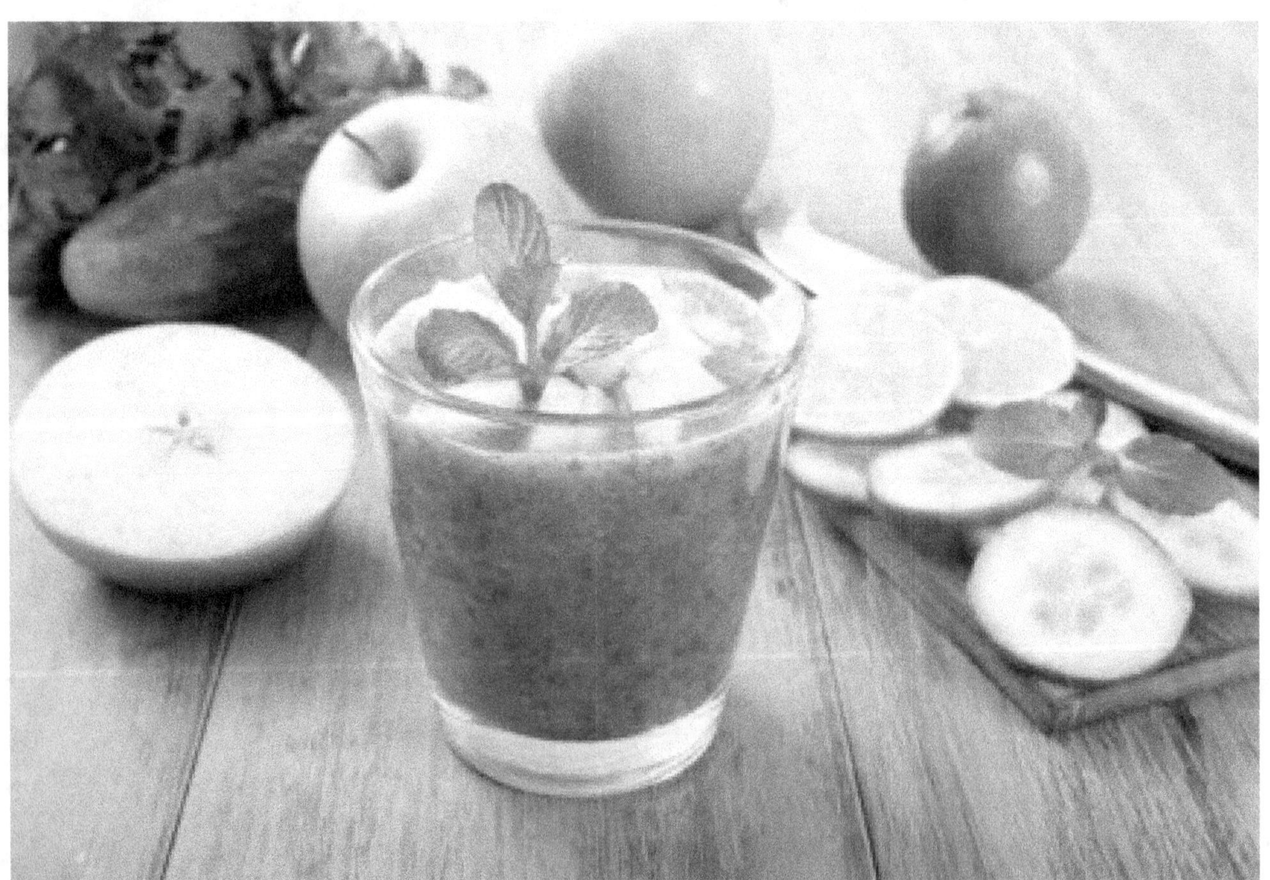

This smoothie can be a healthy replacement for breakfast or lunch. It has enough protein to last you till your next meal. Drink it instead of having rice or bread and the results will be amazing.

Ingredients:
1) Coconut water - 1 cup
2) Baby spinach - 2 large handfuls
3) 1 Fuji apple
4) 1 Pear
5) Plant-based protein powder - 1 scoop

Remove the core of the pear and apple. First, blend spinach in coconut water and then mix in the fruit. You can use simple apple if you don't have Fuji apple.

Spinach Blueberry Smoothie:

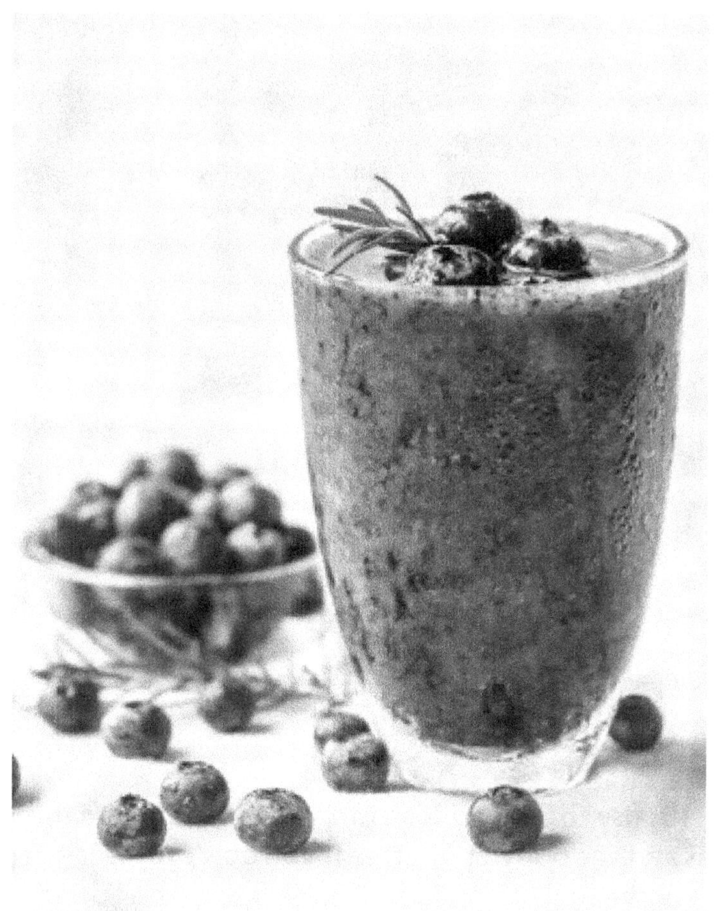

Stocked with minerals and vitamins, spinach and kiwi are good greens to use if you want to lose a few pounds. You don't like the unpleasant taste of spinach? Just add blueberries to mask it and you will get yourself an inviting smoothie.

Ingredients:
1) Frozen spinach - 2 cups
2) 4 mint leaves
3) Blueberries - 2 cups
4) Coconut water – 1 cup
5) One ripe kiwi
6) Ice cubes - 1 cup

Whirl everything in a blender and savor a refreshing smoothie.

Spinach and Yoghurt Smoothie:

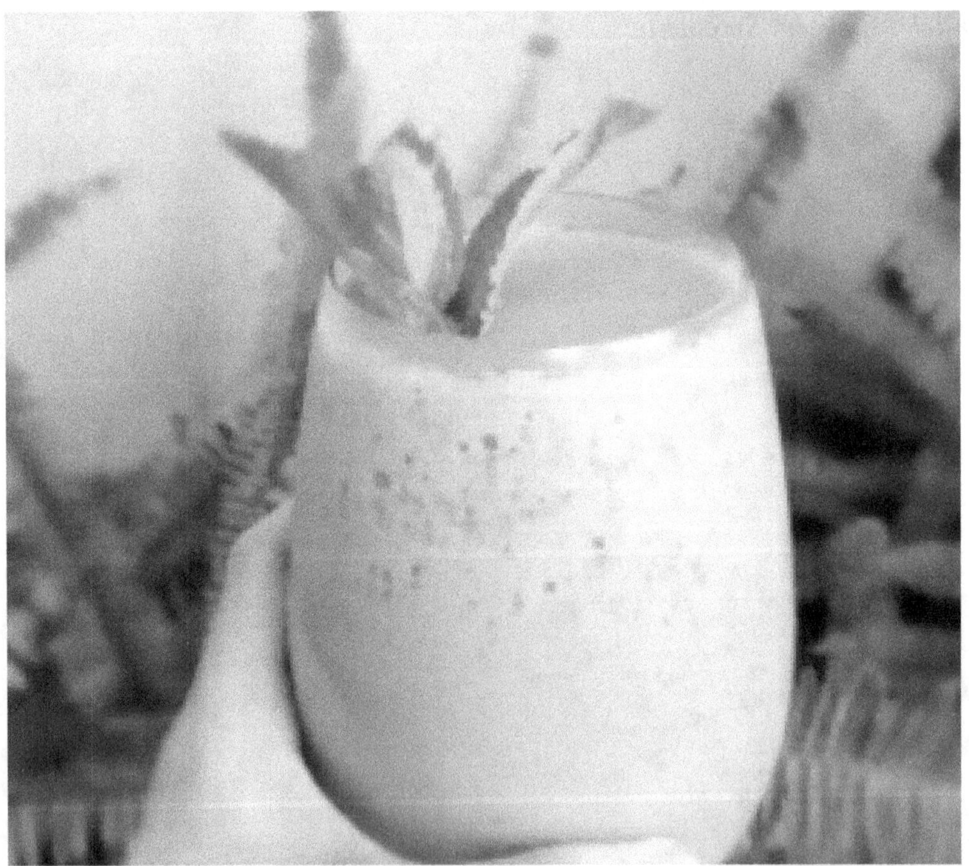

Raw spinach is a powerhouse that provides a range of vitamins and minerals that are important for the skin, bones and the body. It's better if you don't replace coconut milk with other kinds of milks as it is known to have MCT fats. These fats curb appetite and reduce calorie intake of the body. You need them to lose weight.

Ingredients:
1) Raw spinach – 2 cups
2) Coconut milk – 1 cup
3) Greek yogurt – 1 cup
4) 1 Banana

Put all the ingredients in a blender and blend until the smoothie is smooth and creamy. Use frozen banana or ice cubes to relish the flavor better.

Detox Smoothies

There was a time when green smoothies and detox smoothies were disliked because of their strong taste. It's not the same now because so many delicious fruits and natural sweeteners and flavors are available that you don't even feel much of the greens, except in a healthy way. You have no need to pinch your nose while drinking these delectable detox smoothies. These are one of the most delicious yet very healthy detox smoothie recipes. They are packed with anti-oxidants which neutralize free radicals and cleanse your body. So, experience the richness and flavor of all the ingredients while you give your body what it needs. There you go with some super-doper recipes!

Pineapple Detox Smoothie:

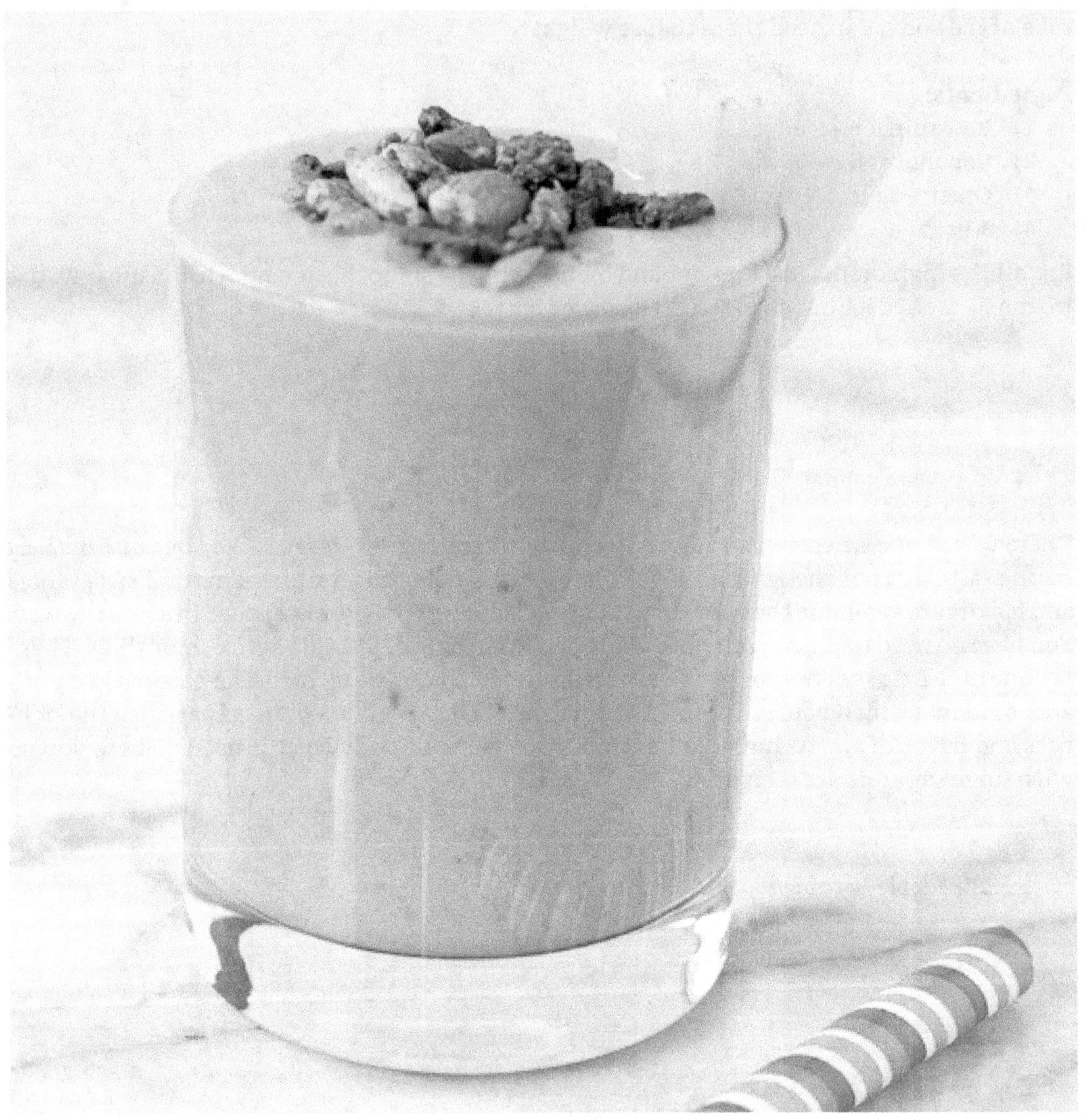

A smoothie with pineapples is bound to be delicious and loaded with nutrients. It has vitamin C, an antioxidant, which strengthens the immune system. Amazingly, it also reduces wrinkles and fine lines. Ladies, you should drink it just for that reason alone.

Ingredients:
1) Pineapple (cut into cubes) - 1 cup
2) Pitted and peeled avocado – 1/2 cup
3) Spinach leaves - 1 cup
4) 1 banana
5) Ginger – 1/2 tsp
6) Almond milk - 1 cup

Blend finely to make a creamy smoothie. Then, enjoy this tasty cleansing smoothie to your heart's content.

Cilantro Ginger Smoothie

Ingredients:

1) Fresh spinach - 1 cup
2) Pineapple chunks – 1/2 cup
3) Banana slices – 1/2 cup
4) One green apple
5) Fresh ginger – 1/2 tsp
6) Lime juice - 1 tbsp.
7) Water or orange juice – 1/2 cup
8) Cilantro - one handful

Give everything a spin in the blender and voila! You have got yourself a detox smoothie. Freeze the banana and pineapple beforehand if you want your smoothie cold.

Nut Detox Smoothie

A good detox smoothie requires three basic things: proteins, vegetables and fruit. With a banana, spinach and almond milk, you will get all the three things needed to remove toxins from your body. The reasons to use almond milk instead of normal milk is that it is free of any harmful bacteria and it's high in protein. It's better to not utilize dairy products when trying to cleanse your body and lose weight.

Ingredients:

1) Fresh Spinach or kale - 2 cups
2) Unsweetened almond milk - ½ cup

3)   Frozen banana - 1
4)   Almond butter - 1 tbsp.

Blend everything and serve fresh. This almond smoothie is known to give a protein boost and the antioxidants come from leafy greens.

Green Citrus Smoothie

Citrus fruits like oranges are popular as detox fruits because they improve liver's ability to detox harmful substances. This not only removes toxins from our body but also keeps our liver healthy and functioning.

Ingredients:
1)   1 Peeled orange
2)   Spinach - 1 cup
3)   Half a banana (fresh/frozen)
4)   Unsweetened coconut water – 3/4 cup
5)   Lemon juice (from a half peeled lemon)

First, blend the orange, spinach and coconut water together until smooth. Subsequently, add in the rest. Blend and savor this orange delicacy.

Superfood Apple Smoothie

Avocado is a superfood brimming with nutrients that help to dilate blood vessels and demolish fatty substances that cause cholesterol. The glutathione in avocado also supports the liver in the difficult process of detoxification.

Ingredients:

1)   Half a sliced avocado
2)   Chopped apple - 1
3)   Apple juice - 1 ½ cup
4)   Spinach or kale (fresh) - 2 cups
5)   Water - as required for the right consistency

When avocado is blended with apple, this smoothie drink can boost the detox process and most definitely makes you slim. What more do you want from a smoothie? Try it out!

Mango Detox Smoothie

If you are not a fan of putting greens in your smoothies, try combining spinach with mangoes. You will love the sweetness of mango and get all the nutritional value from spinach and almond milk.

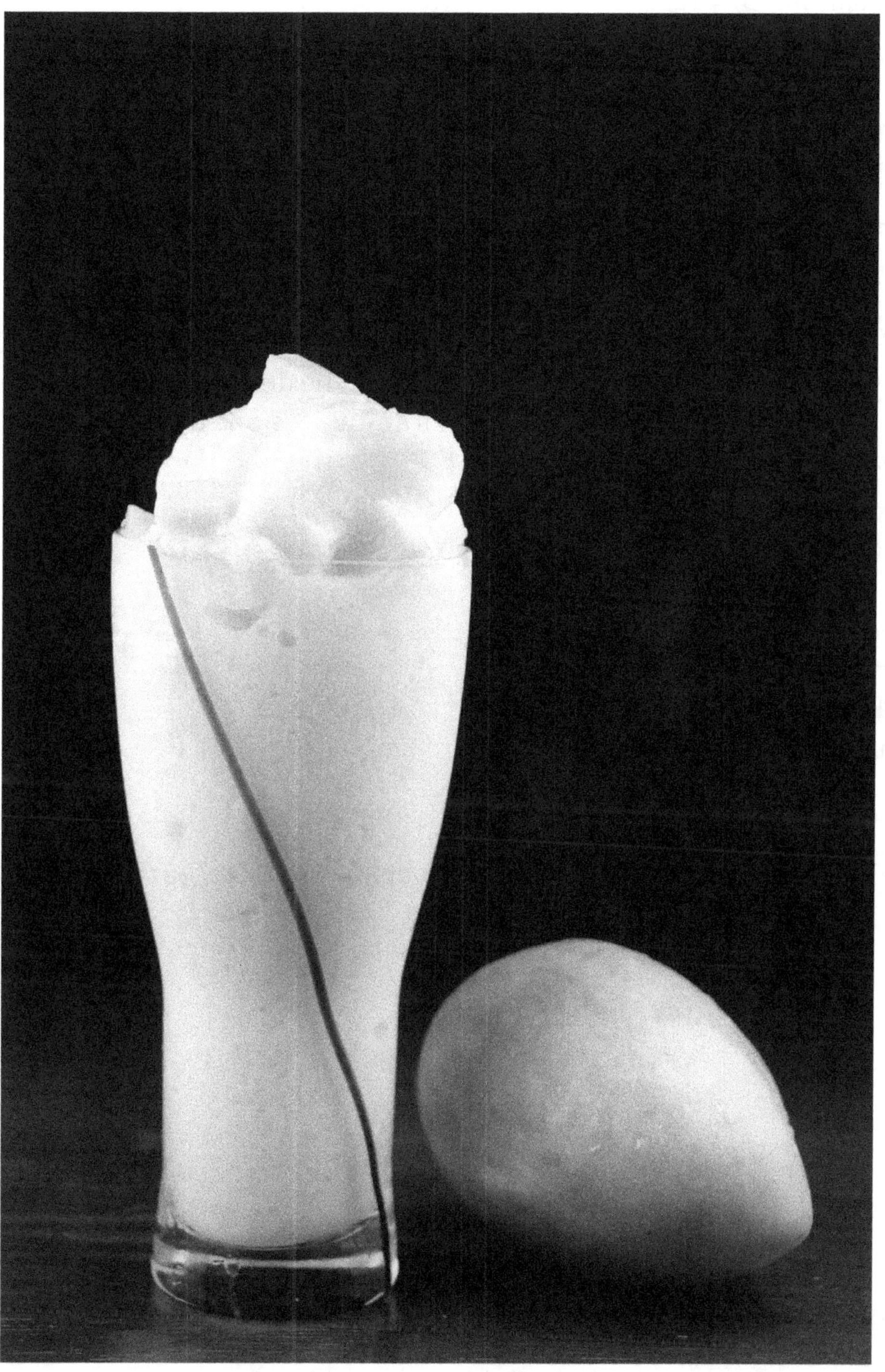

Ingredients:
1) Mango cubes (frozen) – 1/2 cup
2) Baby spinach (fresh) - 1 cup
3) Banana - 1
4) Almond milk – 3/4 cup

Blend everything together to drink this sweet mango smoothie. But start by blending spinach and almond milk. Then add the mango chunks and banana. Drink this delightful smoothie whenever you like!

Collard Oats Smoothie

With collard greens, you can have fabulous skin along with a happy tummy. This smoothie will control your blood sugar level and cholesterol. The dense fiber fruits such as apple and banana will provide you with minerals and vitamins. It's one of the most delicious detox smoothies ever!

Ingredients:

1) One peeled banana
2) Collard greens - 1 ½ cups
3) One sliced apple
4) Cinnamon - 1 tsp
5) Oats - 3 tbsps.
6) Water - 1 cup

Make yourself a healthy detox smoothie with banana and oats. Both are loaded with nutrients.

Strawberry Beets Detox Smoothie

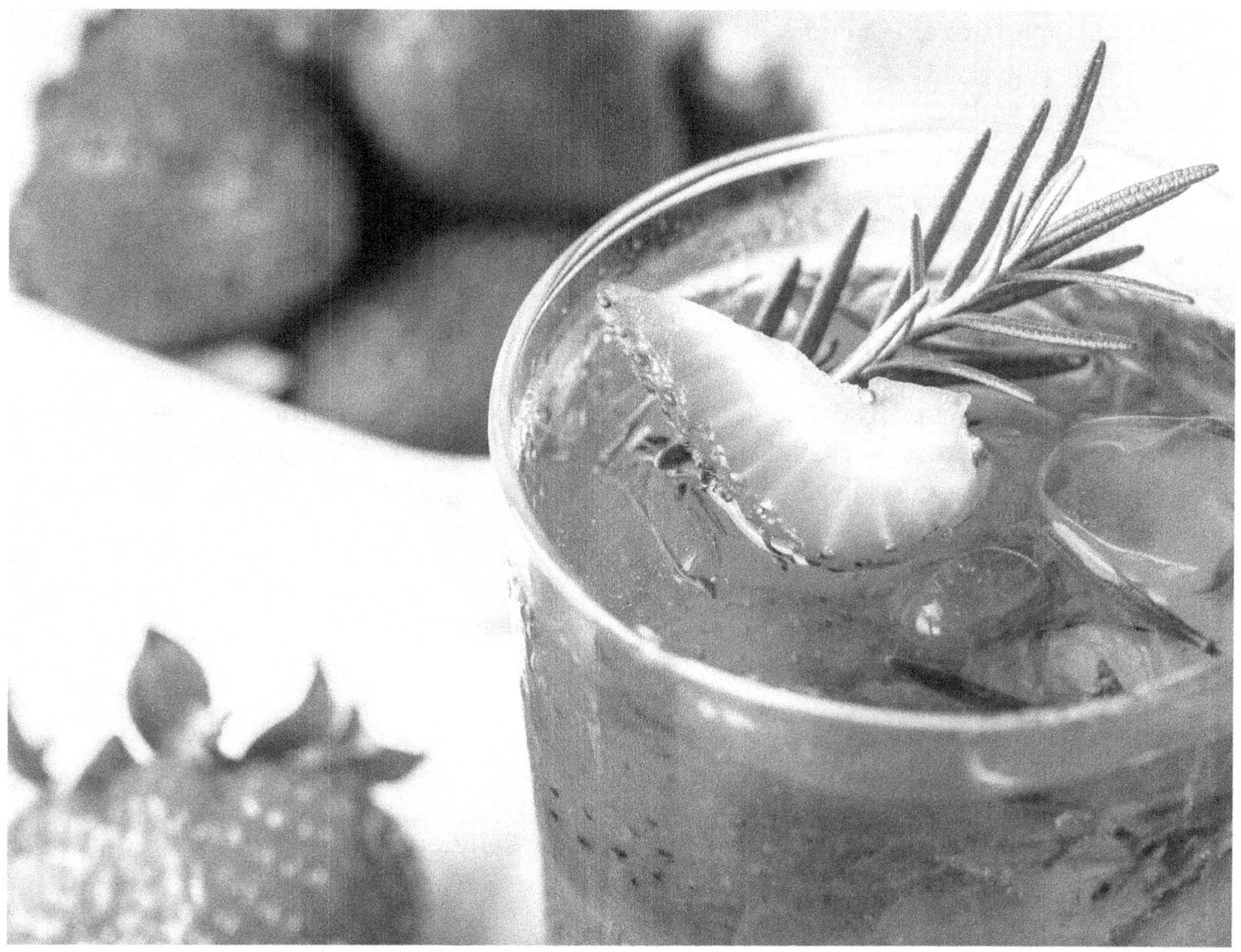

The work of detoxification is in the hands of liver and it is overworked. One way to lessen the burden of liver and boost its cleaning abilities is to drink beetroot detox smoothie. When your liver is working effectively, then not only will you feel better, but your hormones, energy and cholesterol levels will also be maintained properly.

Ingredients:
1) One small red beet
2) Strawberries (frozen) - 1 cup
3) Baby spinach - 1 cup
4) Half avocado
5) 1 green apple

6) Pineapple (frozen) - 1 cup
7) Lemon juice - 1 tbsp.
8) Coconut water - 1 cup

Peel the apple, avocado and the beet. Dice them and blend for 30 to 40 seconds until smoothie is creamy.

Banana Pineapple detox smoothie

This smoothie is super healthy and delicious with tons of nutrients which have antioxidant, anti-inflammatory and disease fighting properties in addition to the promotion of weight loss. Moreover, the calcium in spinach strengthens bones and enriches blood. It is also an excellent drink for aiding digestion.

Ingredients:
1) Pineapple - 1 cup
2) 1 apple
3) 1 banana
4) Spinach - 2 cups
5) Water - 1 cup

Blend all the ingredients smoothly and try out this delicious and easy detox smoothie to help you out!

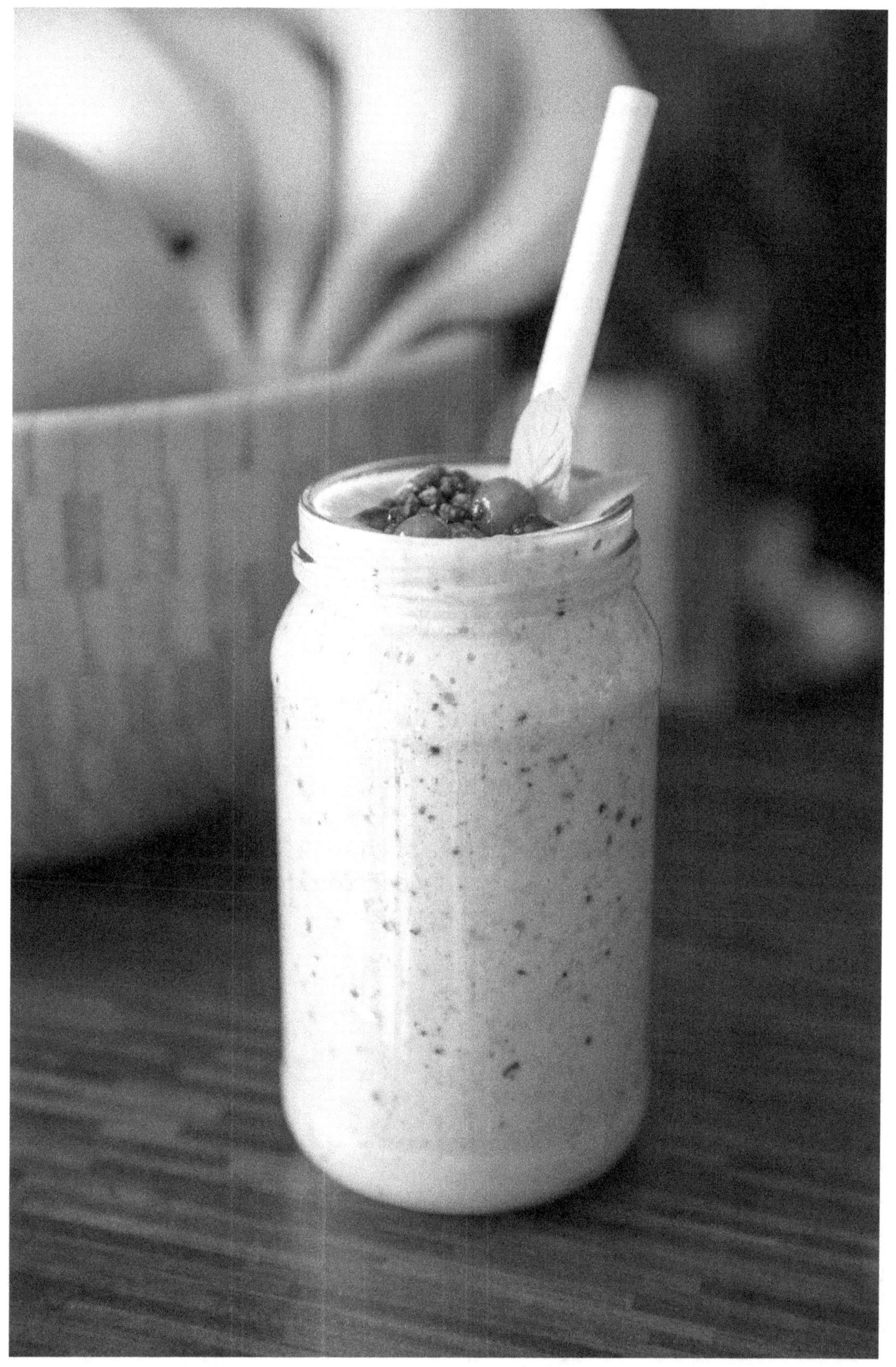

Detox Smoothie Recipe with Avocado

Avocado detox smoothies are super healthy with a blend of potassium, vitamins B and C, folate and many more. It is great for the heart, joints, and eyes and also promotes weight loss. So, this delicious smoothie packs tons of healthy stuff for you.

Ingredients:

1) Apple juice - 1 ½ cups
2) Kale or spinach -2 cups
3) 1 apple
4) Half avocado

Blend it nice and smooth and sip this healthy drink at least once a week to keep yourself healthy and strong.

Strawberry Banana Detox Smoothie with Kale

Kale is called "superfood" as it is the best source of vitamin K. Due to the addition of banana and strawberries in this smoothie, it is not only delicious but also an antioxidant drink. It also aids in digestion, strengthens heart and boosts energy.

Ingredients:

1) 1 banana
2) 1 cup strawberries (fresh or frozen)
3) 1 cup yogurt
4) 1 cup kale (chopped)
5) 1 cup ice

This is a dream drink for all fruit lovers. Blend it nice and smooth and try out this cool and delicious drink.

Banana and Apple Oatmeal Smoothie

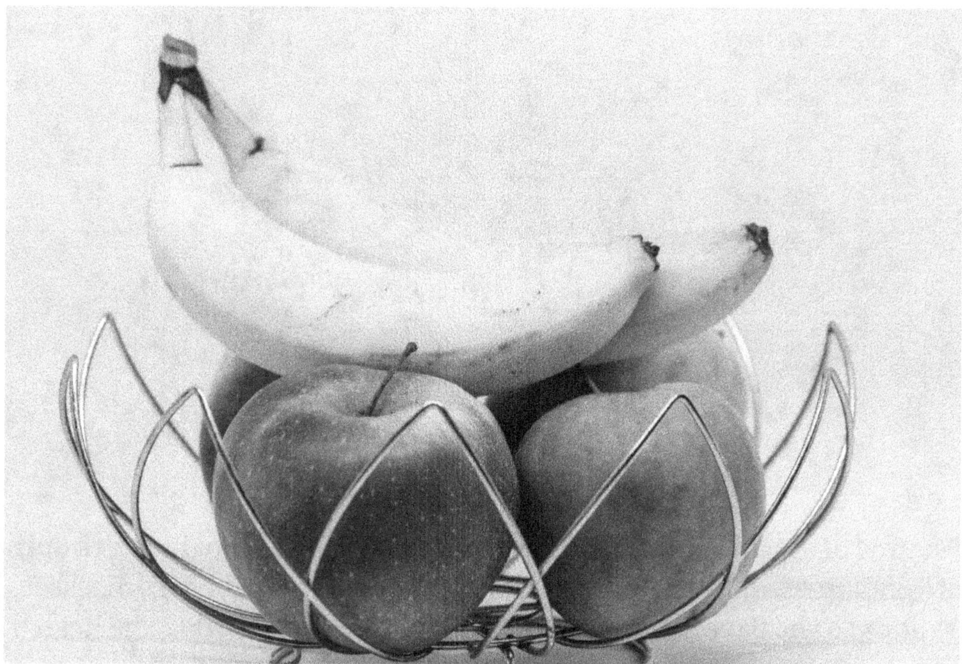

This smoothie is an excellent recipe for breakfast as it is not only healthy and nutritious but also very tasty. As the saying goes, "An apple a day keeps the doctor away", it is an antioxidant, anti-inflammatory, good for heart and blood, lowers cholesterol and promotes weight loss. It contains vitamins, iron, potassium and magnesium. It keeps your stomach and skin both healthy and happy.

Ingredients:

1) Collard greens – 1 cup
2) 1 chopped apple
3) 1 peeled banana
4) Oats – 3 tbsp.
5) Cinnamon – 1 tbsp.
6) Water – 1 cup
7) Ice – 1 cup

Blend the ingredients nice and smooth in a blender. Add ice to make it cool and fresh for a good start to the day!

Greens Pineapple and Orange Smoothie

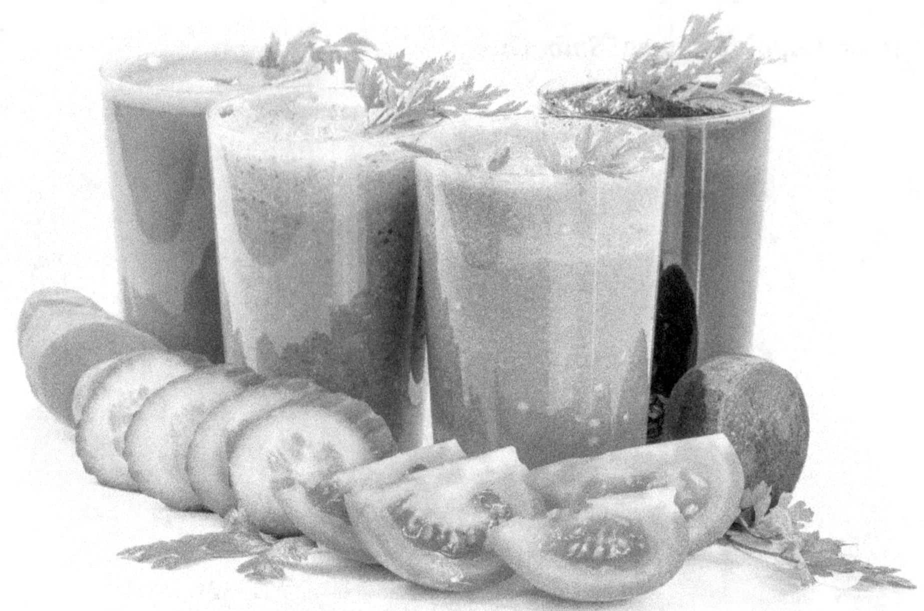

Spinach is a source of vitamins, fiber and minerals. Having a smoothie with spinach is a rich source of antioxidants which reduces the risk of cancer, eye and heart diseases. Addition of certain fruits adds to the flavor and texture of the smoothie as well as the health benefits.

Ingredients:
1)   Pineapple – 1/4 cup
2)   1 peeled orange
3)   1 cup spinach
4)   1 tbsp. flax seeds
5)   1 cup water

Blend all the ingredients till smooth. Add ice to make it refreshing in the hot weather.

Sunflower Peppercorn Smoothie

Peppercorns and sunflower seeds help to rid the toxins from the human body. Sunflower seeds have vitamin E which maintains the substance of lipoproteins. These proteins control the amount of fat in the body so they are really important. While, the celery stick contains many anti-inflammatory properties that aid in keeping the body healthy.

Ingredients:
1.   Fresh peppercorns
2.   Mint leaves – a handful
3.   1 Celery stick

4. 1 Kiwi
5. Half avocado
6. A pinch of salt

Peel and dice avocado and kiwi. Add them in a blender and blend. Toss in the celery stick, mint leaves, peppercorns and sunflower seeds and mix until smooth. Serve by topping with grounded peppercorns.

Cranberry Cucumber Smoothie

Try this brilliant cranberry smoothie not only to detox your body but also to keep your kidneys strong. It is rich in vitamin C, E, K, manganese and a large number of phytonutrients which keeps you miles and miles away from urinary tract infection, cardiovascular disease, cancer and dental problems. Say hello to this remarkable smoothie!

Ingredients:

1) Cranberries – half cup
2) 1 cucumber
3) 1 pear
4) 1 apple
5) 1 celery stalk
6) A handful of spinach

Blend spinach, cucumber and celery first. Then add all the fruits and take advantage of this super healthy smoothie.

Energy Boosting Smoothies

If you need to boost your energy, smoothies are a great and instant way of doing that. Don't go for coffee, tea or an artificial energy drink to give you a kick start. Instead go for the healthier options like a nourishing glass of smoothie. In the presence of such energy boosting smoothies you need not worry about your weakening immune system. They are rich in carbohydrates, proteins, calcium, vitamins, minerals and a lot more to increase the energy reserves of your body.

Grapefruit Pineapple Green Smoothie

Grapefruit is a sweet and sour fruit which is high in nutrients but low in calories. So, this smoothie is rich in fiber, folic acid and vitamins. It promotes diet control, weight loss and benefits our immune system and heart. It makes our bones strong and cleans our blood from toxins. It is a good drink for boosting energy.

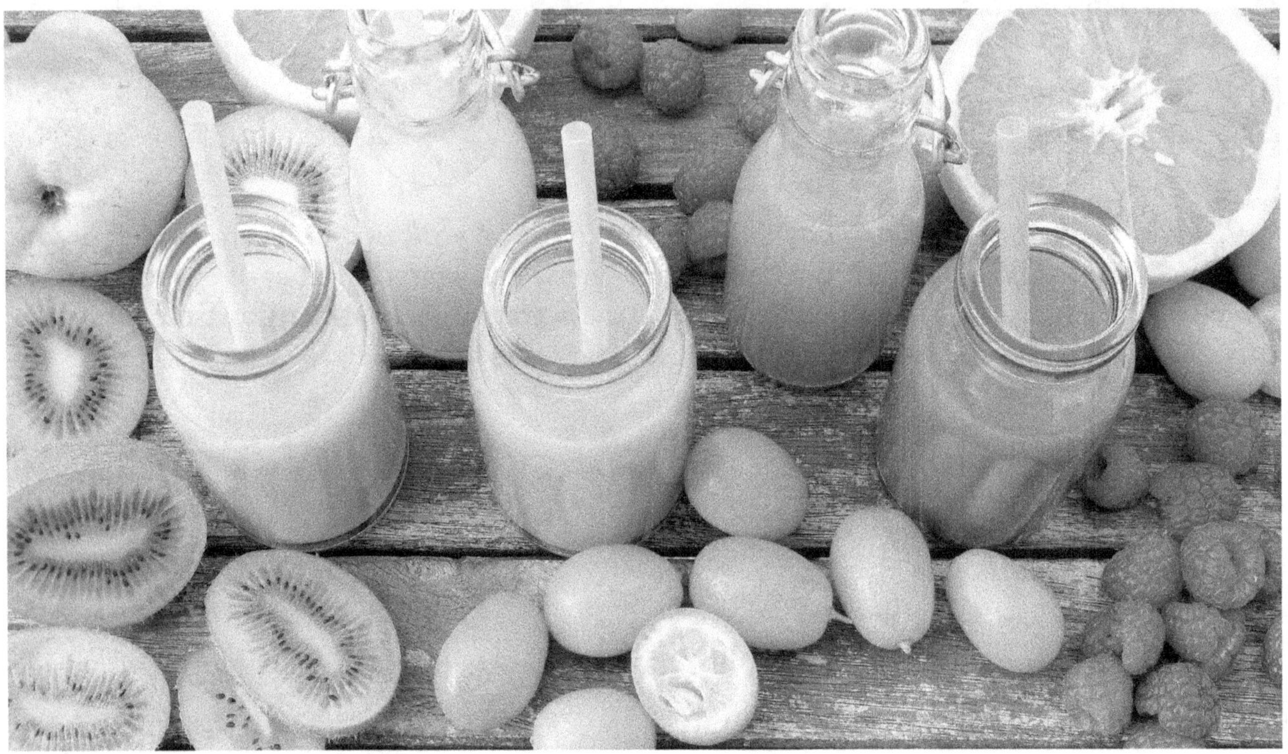

Ingredients:
1) 2 cups fresh spinach
2) 1 cup water
3) 1 grapefruit
4) 2 cups pineapple

Blend spinach, grapefruit and water first and then add pineapple until smooth.

Vegetable and Fruit Smoothie

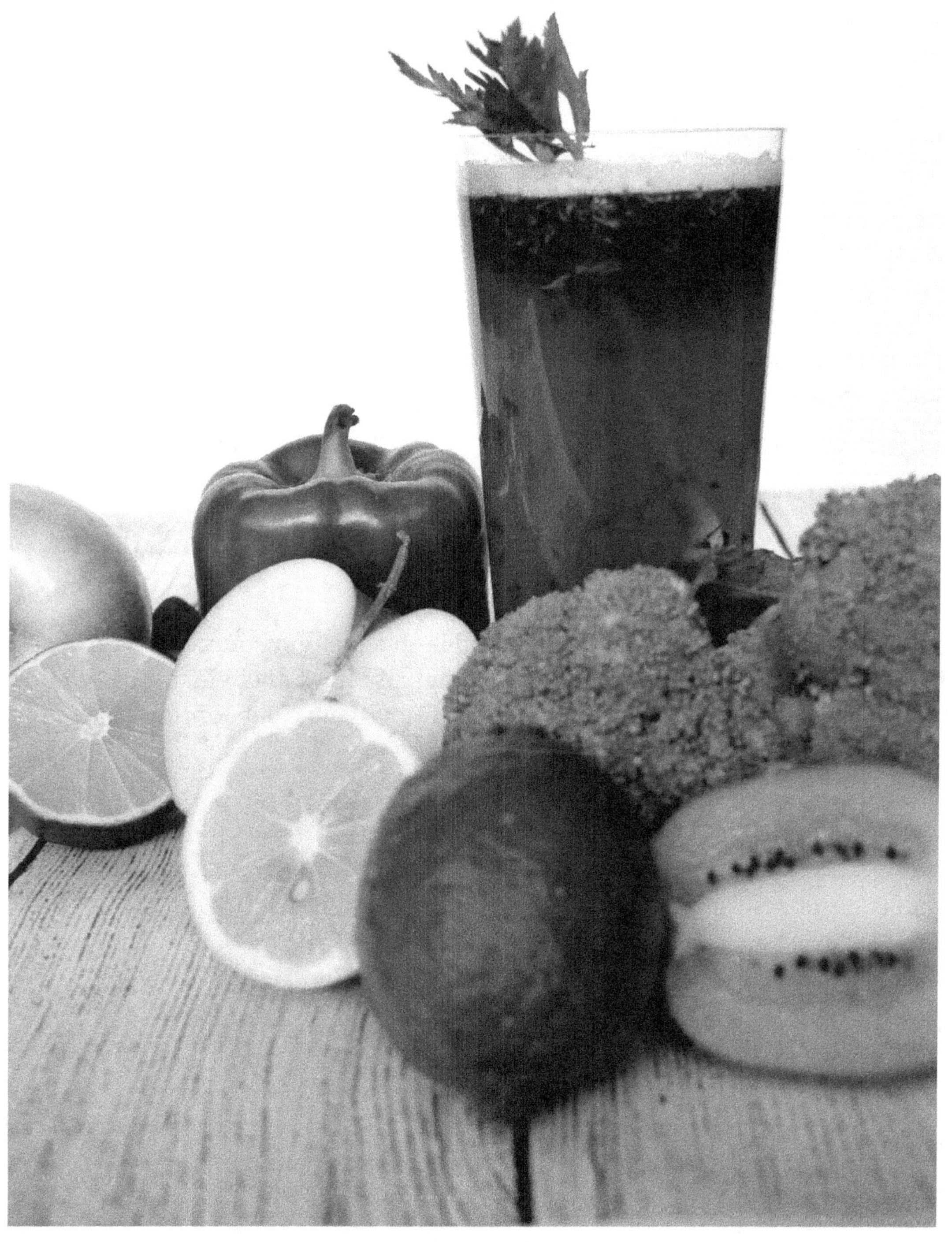

This smoothie is a mixture of various fruits and vegetables giving it a sweet and satisfying taste. This blend

of fruits is high in vitamins and fiber which is very healthy for the body and the ingredients are also super easy to obtain at any market. It is excellent for boosting energy due to the use of so many fruits.

Ingredients

1) Fresh spinach – 1 cup
2) Water – 3/4 cup
3) 1 orange
4) Pineapple – 1/4 cup
5) Mango – 1/4 cup
6) Sliced banana – 1/2 cup

Blend spinach, water and oranges first. Then add remaining ingredients and blend until smooth.

Green Vegetable Smoothie

This recipe is a mixture of green vegetables and is an excellent source of vitamin C, antioxidants and dietary fiber. It promotes weight loss and digestion and is favorable for both health and beauty. Since raw vegetables are used, the amount of nutrient content is very high which helps fight against various diseases and boosts energy.

Ingredients:

1) Half cucumber in small pieces
2) 2 ribs celery
3) 1 pear (peeled and cut in chunks)
4) Half apple (peeled and cut into pieces)
5) 1 lemon
6) 3 cups kale (chop into small pieces)
7) 1 cup baby spinach
8) Half bunch parsley
9) Half cup distilled water

Place apple, lemon juice, pear, celery, cucumber in a high powered blender and blend properly. Add green vegetables and blend until smooth. Add water and blend until thoroughly combined.

Natural Energy Smoothie

This smoothie has powerful medicinal properties. It improves brain function, lowers cholesterol and blood pressure and also has antioxidant properties. It makes you not only fit but also beautiful. The ingredients especially coconut oil and lemon juice are excellent for moisturizing skin. They slow aging and make a person look youthful and fresh, smart and pretty.

Ingredients

1) 2 cups baby kale
2) 2 cups of green tea
3) 2 bananas
4) 1 cup blueberries
5) 2 tbsp. Coconut oil
6) 1 tbsp. ginger root
7) 2 tbsp. chia seeds
8) 1 tbsp. lemon juice

First blend kale and green tea and then add remaining ingredients and make a smooth puree. Don't forget to try this energy boosting smoothie!

Chocolate Smoothie

Cocoa powder is rich in polyphenols which improves blood flow to the brain and brain function. It is a delight in improving the mood and easing depression. Children all love it so let your kids have a taste of this yummy and healthy drink. Rich in vitamins and antioxidant properties, this smoothie aids in weight loss, digestion and boosting energy.

Ingredients:
1) 1 cup spinach
2) 1 cup almond milk
3) 1 cup strawberries
4) 1 banana

5) 2 tbsp. cocoa powder

Make a puree of spinach and almond milk. Add fruit and cocoa powder and blend until smooth. Have this drink on busy and depressing days to boost your energy and mood!

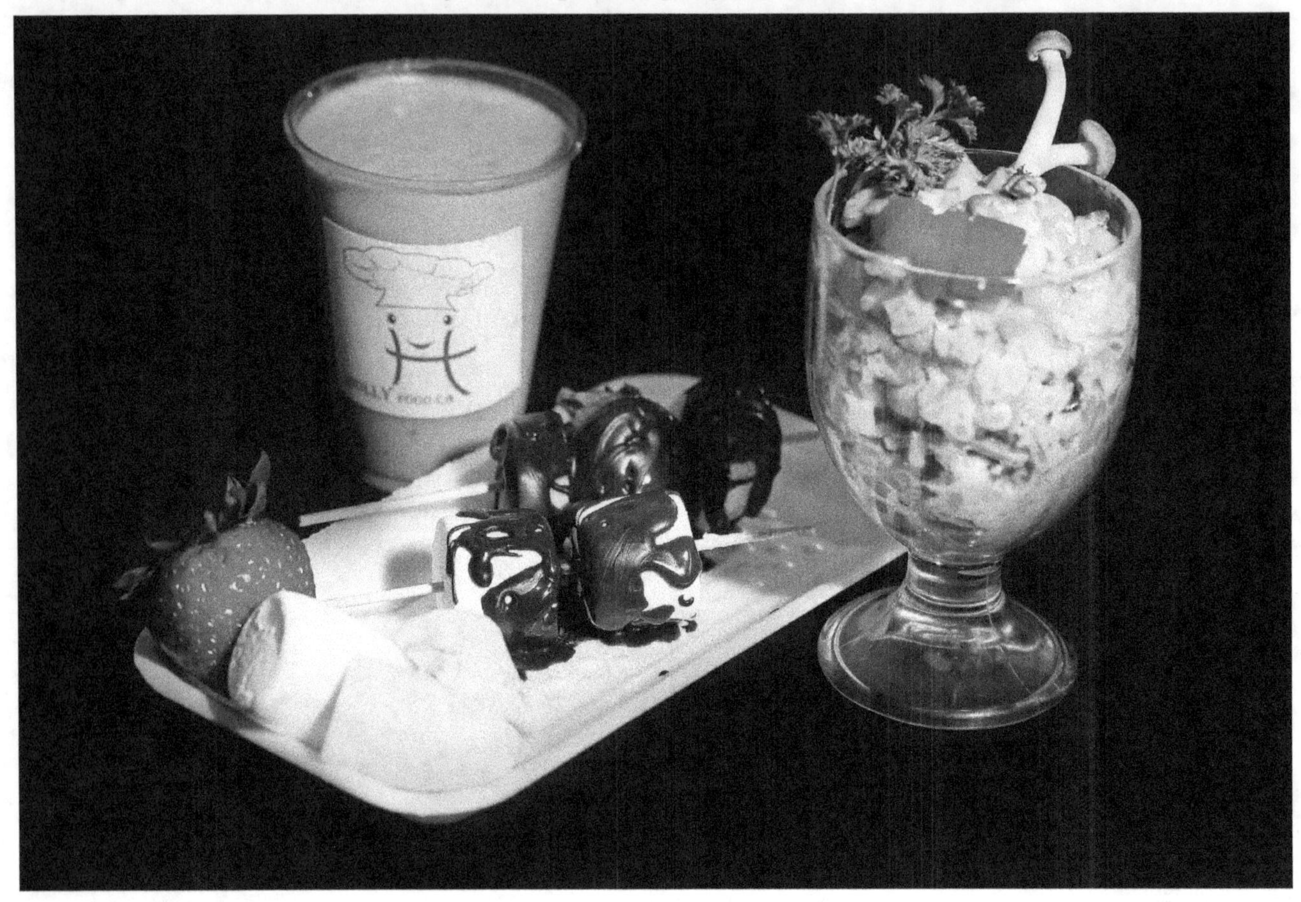

Cranberry Smoothie

Cranberries are winter fruit and are mostly ready for harvesting during autumn but are also available all year round in frozen form. They are rich in antioxidants, fiber, vitamins, manganese, copper, phytonutrients etc. They improve urinary tract and gut health thus, preventing infection. They boost the immune system and energy. It is great that they are low in calories and sugar. Hence, a person does not need to worry about gaining weight.

Ingredients:
1) Fresh spinach - 1 cup
2) Cranberries – 1/2 cup

3) 1 orange
4) Water - 1 cup
5) Half banana

Make a puree of spinach and water in a blender. Add fruit and blend again until smooth and creamy delight forms. Sip this drink all year round and keep yourself healthy and energetic!

Kale Pineapple Smoothie

This recipe is super easy and the ingredients are available at any supermarket. It takes only five ingredients to assemble the whole recipe and a healthy and nutritious smoothie will be ready in five minutes. It is rich in fiber, antioxidants, vitamin C and K and monounsaturated fatty acids which are good for protection against many diseases.

Ingredients:
1) 1 cup kale leaves
2) Chopped Pineapple – 1/4 cup
3) Half avocado
4) Water or coconut water – 1 cup
5) Coconut oil - 1 tbsp.

Blend kale leaves in coconut water. You can add a teaspoon of matcha green tea for extra energy boost or half cup unsweetened Greek yogurt for creamy texture. You can even replace avocado with a banana. Blend all the ingredients at a high speed in a blender until smooth. Add ice if you want to.

Peanut Smoothie

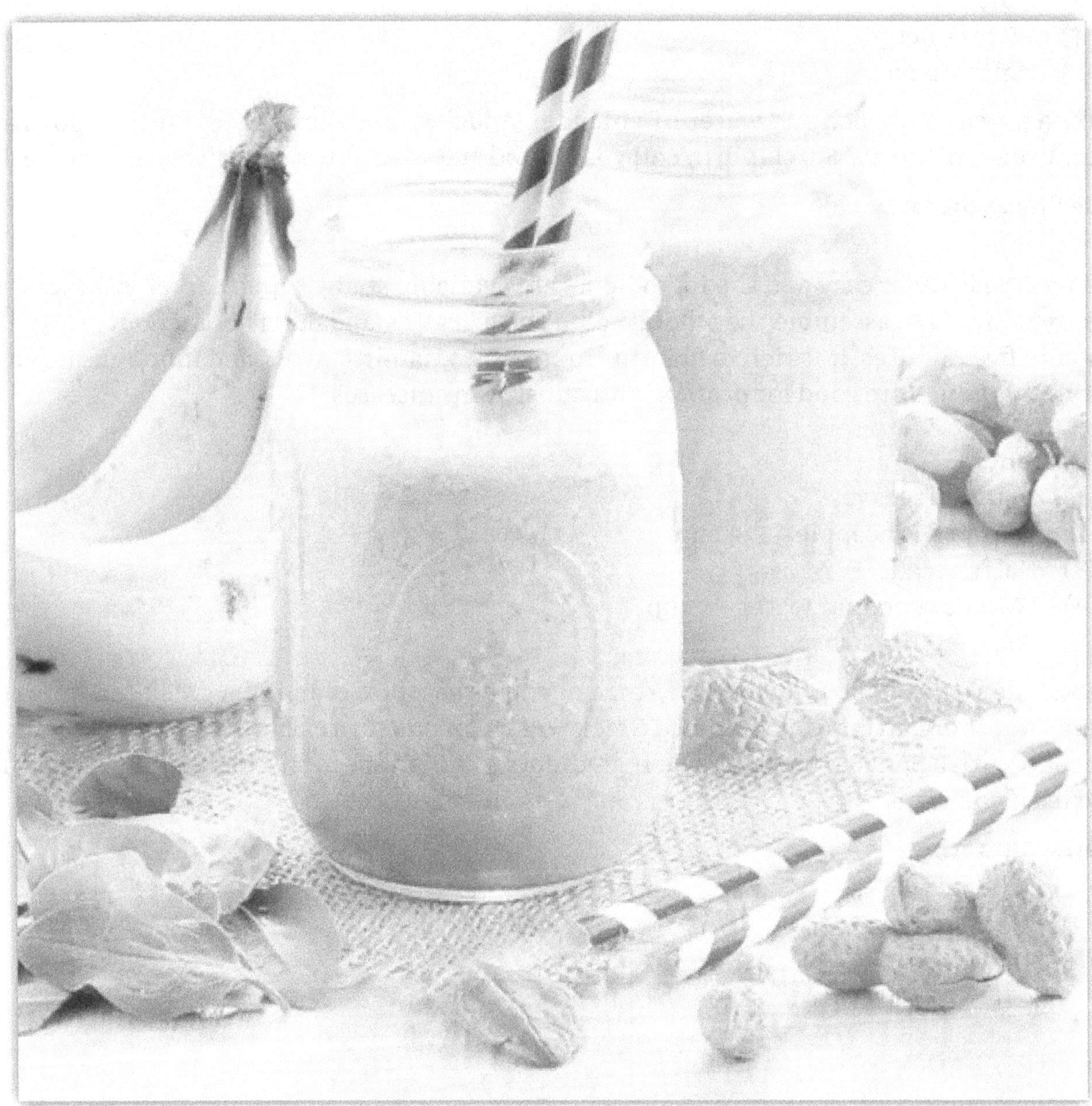

Made with peanuts and peanut butter, this smoothie provides you with instant energy as both of these ingredients are the source of high energy monounsaturated and polyunsaturated fatty acids that boost the body's energy level. For those who don't like breakfast, this smoothie acts as a satisfying morning drink. Drinking it before and after exercise helps the muscles and body's energy level.

Ingredients:
1) Peanuts - 2 tbsp.

2)   1 handful of spinach
3)   1 banana
4)   Almond milk - 1 cup
5)   Peanut butter - 1 bsp
6)   6 large ice cubes

Blend the ingredients until smooth. It's for peanut lovers because this drink taste just like peanuts!

Berry and Chia Smoothie

The addition of chia seeds in this smoothie makes it an energy drink. Chia seeds are a rich source of omega three fatty acids that help to boost energy for a long time and is even helpful in burning calories. The smoothie is hearty and healthy and is sure to fill you up with nutrients and protect you against

diseases.

Ingredients:

1)   Chia seeds - 2 tbsp.
2)   1 orange
3)   Strawberries - 1 cup
4)   Spinach - 2 cups
5)   Blueberries - 1 cup
6)   Water - 1 ½ cups

Blend spinach, chia seed and water first to dissolve the seeds. Add fruits later and blend again. Drink this hearty smoothie that fills your tummy and keeps you energetic.

Nutty Green Smoothie

Nuts are rich sources of protein, healthy fats, vitamins, fiber and folic acid. A smoothie that includes nut butter and nut milk is a dream come true for nut lovers and vegetarians alike for they gain protein without meat. This smoothie is dairy free, reduces risk of disease, and it is low in calories and sugar. In addition to that, it is a natural energy booster and you won't get hungry till your next meal.

Ingredients:
1) Spinach - Half cup
2) Half frozen banana
3) Nut milk - 1 cup
4) Nut butter - 1 to 2 tbsp.
5) Half cup rolled oats
6) Blueberries – 1/4 cup

Blend all ingredients until smooth. Feel free to add ice if you like your smoothies cold. Drink it when it reaches your desired consistency and temperature.

Energy Boosting Fruit Smoothie

This smoothie is a mixture of powerful antioxidants, anti-inflammatory properties as well as proteins that are building blocks of our body. Aside from strengthening the body and boosting energy, this smoothie aids anemic patients, have anti-cancer properties and lowers blood pressure. Drinking this smoothie will manage your health issues and keep other diseases away from you. Plus, it will keep you strong and energized.

Ingredients:
1) 2 handfuls of spinach
2) Lemon juice - 1 tbsp.
3) Almond butter - 1 tbsp.
4) Almond milk - 1 cup
5) Blueberries – 1/4 cup
6) Half banana
7) Chia seed - 1 tbsp.

Blend the ingredients properly until smooth. Adjust its consistency, sweetness and temperature as desired. This is a perfect way to start your morning in a refreshing and healthy way for all men and women!

Flax Meal Smoothie

This smoothie recipe is great for gut health. It has powerful omega 3 fatty acid which makes it an excellent energy booster. The smoothie also contains potassium and fiber and has many medicinal properties. Using kale as green vegetable is an excellent choice as it is a superfood packed with all the essential nutrients to build and strengthen the body.

Ingredients:

1. 2 dates
2. Flax meal - 1 tbsp.
3. Chopped kale - 2 cups
4. Sliced banana - 2 cups
5. Orange juice - 1 ½ cups

Use frozen banana to enhance the flavor. Using half teaspoon of fresh grated ginger is optional for people who like it. Put kale and orange juice in a high speed blender. Blend and add all the ingredients until it's smooth and delicious. Body builders should use it before or after exercise for boosting energy.

Fruity Green Smoothie

The recipe includes banana, pineapple and mango all of which are naturally sweet fruits. It is a clever way to add greens to your daily smoothies to add to the health benefits an ordinary drink provides. Clearly rich with nutrients, vitamins and minerals, this smoothie is also a natural energy booster. A great thing about this recipe is that all the ingredients are easily available.

Ingredients:
1) Frozen pineapple chunks – 1/2 cup
2) Frozen mango chunks – 1/2 cup
3) Baby spinach – 1/2 cup
4) Almond milk – 1/2 cup
5) 1 small sliced banana

The spinach leaves should be fresh and mango and pineapple unsweetened. First blend almond milk and spinach properly. Add remaining ingredients and repeat the blending process. Serve it cold and enjoy!

Ginger and Turmeric Green Smoothie

Turmeric and ginger both possess antioxidant and anti-inflammatory properties. Using them in the smoothie reduces the threat of nasty winter colds and let you enjoy the weather wholeheartedly. It is good for digestion and boosts the body's energy. Ginger and turmeric have been used in Asia for centuries to heal wounds. Now, use these magic ingredients to improve your health.

Ingredients:

1) 2 oranges
2) A handful of spinach or kale
3) 1 lemon
4) 2 inches fresh ginger
5) 2 small pieces of turmeric
6) Water - 1 cup

First blend ginger, turmeric and greens in water. Then blend in oranges and lemon. Add 4-5 ice cubes to make it cold. You can also use mint leaves to make it more refreshing.

Strawberry and Tofu Green Smoothie

This drink includes a variety of ingredients such as Greek yogurt, tofu, strawberries, and chia seeds. All of these are excellent health remedies. They contain proteins, fats, vitamins, and fiber. They are good for heart, lowering blood sugar, blood pressure, cholesterol and protect against stroke. This smoothie improves gut health and protects against bacteria. It is a great energy booster due to rich amount of nutrients used to make this superb drink.

Ingredients:

1) Frozen strawberries - 2 cups
2) Baby spinach - 2 cups
3) Chia seeds - 2 tbsp.
4) Greek yogurt - 1 cup
5) Organic tofu – 1/2 cup
6) Almond milk - 1 cup

There is no better combination than almond milk and Greek yoghurt for making your smoothie super creamy and rich in proteins. Combine the ingredients in a blender until smooth. A perfect remedy for boosting energy in hot days will be ready in barely five minutes. Fill the glass and enjoy!

◆ ◆ ◆

Wrapping Up

Congratulations on taking the first step and making this far in your health journey. Remember that weight loss is both a journey and a learning process. A phrase that is used often "Knowledge is power" is actually true for dealing with our own bodies and health. The more we know about food, the better understanding we develop when it comes to making smart choices for our health. It ultimately has a huge impact on our lives. Now is the time to plan ahead and think how you want to be in the future. Whether you want to look back after 10 years with regrets in your mind or you want to be proud of making right choices.

You only get one life and you want to live it with passion and full energy. Avoid these mistakes and be that person who is confident and loving.

- Making decisions that harm you
- Not loving yourself
- Not focusing on self-improvement and growth
- Not caring for yourself
- Letting others to make decisions for you
- Not learning to excel at anything
- Giving up
- Worrying too much about everything
- Not doing what you really want
- I'll do it tomorrow

You are strong and you can do better and even excel in life. All it takes is self-love and courage. Instead, do the opposite of these regrettable mistakes.

- ➤ Love yourself because it is the heart and soul of everything you do in life.
- ➤ Take action and strive to improve yourself.
- ➤ Start caring for yourself and only then you can care for others.
- ➤ Make your own decisions
- ➤ Keep going
- ➤ Don't worry! Everything will be okay!
- ➤ Follow your heart
- ➤ Start Today!

If you are reading this, it means you care and you have gone through the hard part. You have gained power over your body, your decisions and your life! The information in this book provides you all the tools, tips and techniques to materialize your dream of a healthy and beautiful body. Experience the powerful impacts of 10 Day Green Smoothie Cleanse and share your story with others. Celebrate your success and help others start this health journey. Go ahead and make yourself slim, smart, healthy and happy!